Total Recovery

Total RECOVERY

SOLVING THE MYSTERY OF CHRONIC PAIN AND DEPRESSION

How We GET SICK	Why We STAY SICK	How We Can RECOVER

Dr. Gary Kaplan, D.O.
with Donna Beech

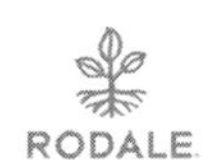

Although the case studies throughout the book have been dramatized for narrative purposes, none of the medical facts have been changed. Names and identifying details have been altered to protect the anonymity of my patients. In some cases, patient composites have been used for that reason. The symptoms, treatments, and results have all been conveyed precisely as they occurred.

Rodale books may be purchased for business or promotional use or for special sales.
For information, please write to:
Special Markets Department, Rodale Inc., 733 Third Avenue, New York, NY 10017

Printed in the United States of America
Rodale Inc. makes every effort to use acid-free ♾, recycled paper ♲.

Book design by Christina Gaugler

Library of Congress Cataloging-in-Publication Data is on file with the publisher.

ISBN 978-1-62336-275-1 trade hardcover

Distributed to the trade by Macmillan

2 4 6 8 10 9 7 5 3 1 hardcover

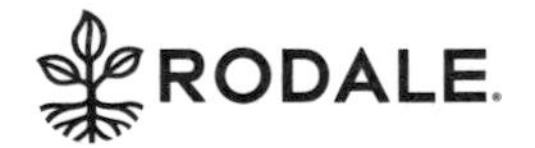

We inspire and enable people to improve their lives and the world around them.
rodalebooks.com

FOR MY PARENTS

The blessing of their love and support cannot be measured.

Contents

Introduction

THINKING ABOUT ZEBRAS

WHAT HAD TO HAPPEN FIRST

A hundred times every day I remind myself that my inner and outer life are based on the labors of other men . . . and that I must exert myself in order to give in the same measure as I have received and am still receiving.

Albert Einstein

My job is to think about zebras.

In medical school, they used to tell us, "When you hear hoofbeats, think horses, not zebras." It's a version of Occam's razor: "The simplest answer is the best." And it's good advice. Swollen lymph nodes and a high fever might be Kawasaki disease, but it's far more likely to be a strep infection.

By the time I see most of my patients, the simplest answers have already been explored. They've already been tested by 8 to 15 specialists from Johns Hopkins, the Mayo Clinic, and other excellent medical centers. If it were a horse, they would've found it.

The patients I see are mysteries: a healthy, athletic 14-year-old boy who plunges into years of excruciating pain after an ACL tear and a flood in the basement; a high-powered consultant for international conglomerates who suddenly finds herself standing in a conference room with 15 executives, a migraine, and no idea how she got there.

My strategy has always been to treat the whole person, not the symptoms. But as a medical scientist, I was convinced that, when patients in chronic pain had a history of emotional, physical, and infectious assaults, all of those assaults must somehow be working together. They were all happening within the ecosystem of the body.

There had to be a single point of origin that connected them all. The question plagued me: *What was the underlying mechanism?*

In the end, I found it. This book tells the story of the clues that led up to that discovery, the *Eureka!* moment when I suddenly understood what we'd been missing, and the aftermath where I confirmed, in patient after patient, that all of their apparently unrelated symptoms actually had a single neurological basis.

It all came back to Occam's razor, after all.

Steve Jobs once said that people who come up with groundbreaking ideas often feel reluctant to take any credit for them. "They just *saw* something," he said. "It seemed obvious to them after a while."[1] Their insights are based on their ability to see a connection based on the experiences they've had. I feel exactly the same way.

All of my education, my patients, my mentors—every experience I've had in medicine and in my own family—had to happen first, or I would never have seen this connection.

PLACEBO AT BEST

In the 1970s, a lot of people were starting to realize that, as impressive as it was, conventional medicine did not have all the answers. Alternative practitioners of every ilk were springing up around the country. People were going to health food stores for vitamin supplements and organic food and getting treatments from chiropractors and acupuncturists, despite the fact that their medical doctors were telling them it was pointless.

From a conventional medical perspective, alternative medical treatments were quackery at worst, placebo at best. Little distinction was made between acupuncture, chiropractic, homeopathy, herbal prescriptions, magnetic therapy, aura cleansing, and faith healing. At the end of World War II, physical therapy carved out a tentative place on the fringes of respectable medicine,[2] but it would be decades before doctors would stop associating massage therapy with hookers and happy endings.

Then, when Richard Nixon went to China in 1971, an amazing thing happened. A *New York Times* correspondent covering President Nixon's historic visit had an emergency appendectomy. James Reston was rushed to the Chinese Anti-Imperialist Hospital.[3] At first, his treatment was similar to our practices in the West. Doctors gave him a standard injection of Xylocaine and benzocaine to anesthetize the area, though Reston was surprised to be kept awake for the whole surgery. A few nights later, when he complained of pain, things began to seem foreign.

Li Chang-yuan, a doctor of acupuncture at the hospital, was sent to treat him. Reston was slightly reluctant but decided to consider it an experiment. When Reston agreed, the doctor inserted three long, thin needles into his right elbow and below his knees, then manipulated the needles. Within an hour, his pain was gone and never came back.

To his surprise, Reston learned that Professor Li Pang-chi, the medical doctor responsible for his case, had initially been reluctant to accept acupuncture as a viable treatment, too. Despite his reservations, he had come to recognize that "the body is an organic unity, that illness can be caused by imbalances between organs and that stimulation from acupuncture can help restore balance."[4]

In his seminal piece in the *New York Times*, Reston wrote, "It has been suggested that maybe this . . . was a journalistic trick to learn something about needle anesthesia. This is not only untrue, but greatly overrates my gifts of imagination, courage and self-sacrifice. There are many things I will do for a good story, but getting slit open in the night or offering myself as an experimental porcupine is not among them."[5]

If Americans winced, it wasn't for long. What they saw for the first time was a brave journalist subjecting himself to long, thin, strange-looking needles. And then, without the full body blow of narcotics—without so much as a second needling—his postoperative pain went away. When Reston quoted Dr. Hsu Hung-tu as saying, "Diseases have inner and outer causes. The higher nervous system of the brain affects the general physiology,"[6] Americans were listening.

Health-conscious "fitness nuts" in California and elsewhere were already jogging, going to chiropractors, and eating tofu. They had never liked the idea of taking heavy narcotics for pain or general anesthesia for minor surgeries. After Reston's article, they started to become curious about what acupuncture could offer.

Previously, people had believed that acupuncture was either pure bunk or placebo. From a Western medical model, sticking needles into the body made no sense at all. It was laughable. But the counterculture movement at home and abroad was gradually making Americans aware that people from all different ethnicities and backgrounds might actually have something to offer. The white American patriarchy was not the only source of knowledge and authority. Both patients and doctors were beginning to think that either millions of Chinese people had been duped for 2,500 years or there was something to the practice of acupuncture.

At first, when American doctors tried to use the techniques, they got highly unreliable results. Chinese medicine is premised on a network of energy meridians that correspond to different organs. Taking a practical approach, the doctors merely stuck the needles in the designated points, without understanding any of the principles behind the practice. They might as well have tried to take blood by stabbing a syringe into the patient's body at random. Doing acupuncture with a Western approach was just as unlikely to work.

As a result, acupuncture was branded "an experimental medical procedure" in 1978. Under this designation, it could only be performed by authorized doctors under experimental protocols. But by that time, the public was so enthralled with acupuncture that many people went to England, France, or China to study it. I went to Monterey.

OFF ON THE RIGHT FOOT

Internal medicine specialist Hector Prestera, MD, was one of the first physicians in the country to use acupuncture. When I graduated college, I drove to California to meet him and ended up studying acupuncture with him for a year before I went to medical school, expecting to be a neurologist.

As I explain in Chapter 1, that aspiration was doomed from the start. After learning to see the body as a whole, the idea of treating individual symptoms as if they had nothing to do with each other—which Western neurology teaches—was as appalling to me as operating with a blindfold on.

Acupuncture opened my eyes to a different and fascinating way of viewing human health. Its diagnoses sounded vague and poetic. In an effort to become more scientific and precise, Western medicine had long ago abandoned poetry and metaphors. So on the surface, the Chinese meridian system seemed whimsical, perhaps even dangerous.

Because it was looking for patterns of disharmony, rather than discrete dysfunctions, it might identify a "liver disorder" that would never show up on clinical laboratory tests. From a Chinese medicine perspective, premenstrual syndrome, for example, is frequently "a disorder of the liver with an invasion of spleen." This kind of diagnosis understandably might sound like nonsense to Western medical ears. I might have thought so, too, except its effectiveness had given me a profound respect for this point of view.

And yet, in the early days of my training, it was my very understanding of Chinese medicine that constantly brought me back to Western physiology. I could see that it worked in ways that Western medicine was not yet addressing, but I couldn't figure out what that meant from a Western perspective. Driven by the need to find a unifying whole, I ultimately added a number of specialties. I was constantly investigating new techniques, learning to evaluate patients from as many directions as possible, since no medical approach explained everything I was seeing in my practice.

When it came to choosing my residency, the only specialty I could find that came close to treating the whole person was family medicine, so I began a residency at Georgetown University in Washington, DC.

It was 1982. As it happened, Joe Helms, MD, who created the Medical Acupuncture for Physicians program through the UCLA continuing medical education office, also invited me to be one of the first students. His was the first comprehensive acupuncture training program created for physicians in the United States. Eager to learn more about a system that treated the body as a whole, while building a strong foundation in Western medicine, I arranged with my Georgetown residency director to spend part of my elective time training in Dr. Helms's program. The basic program started out as a 3-month commitment. As he continued to build the program, adding advanced training and bringing in master acupuncturists from around the world to teach us, my 3-month commitment turned into 8 years of regular 2,300-mile commutes between coasts.

When a major university like UCLA started training doctors in acupuncture, it was a sign that people were beginning to recognize that this ancient Chinese practice had something significant to contribute to our own impressive achievements in Western medicine. Eventually, my acupuncture work led to my helping to create the American Academy of Medical Acupuncture (AAMA), where I served on the board for 5 years. My involvement in the field was such that I later became president of the Medical Acupuncture Research Foundation (MARF).

THE CUSP OF CHANGE

By the 1990s in America, things were changing. We were on the cusp of exciting new discoveries that would lead us to radically alter our understanding of medicine and the nature of the brain itself.

One of the tools we needed had already been invented. In 1990, Seiji Ogawa, PhD, a research scientist at Bell Laboratories in New Jersey, came up with a way to take images of the brain in action.

Magnetic resonance imaging (MRI) had been providing us with still images of the brain since the 1970s. Positron-emission tomography

(PET) scans (affectionately known as "head shrinkers") with radioactive tracers were used to determine how the organs and tissues in the body were working.[7] With MRI and computerized tomography (CT) scans, doctors had the ability to see the brain to identify tumors and other abnormalities, but not to see how the brain actually worked. Then Ogawa improved on the design. Once he figured out a way to create functional magnetic resonance imaging (fMRI), doctors no longer needed to guess what was going on in the brain. We could see how the brain worked—*live,* for the very first time.

In that same year, the Hubble Telescope was launched into space. It was like turning on a light in a dark room. Astrophysicists, like brain research scientists, could see what they were studying in a completely new way.

Technological breakthroughs in the early 1990s gave us access to an unprecedented magnitude of information about our bodies, our world, and our universe. Soon after the World Wide Web was launched in 1991, search engines were developed to help us sift through vast amounts of data.

With the advent of 24-hour access to such enormous banks of knowledge, startling new medical insights began to emerge. The Human Genome Project was launched at National Institutes of Health (NIH) in 1990. By June 2000, scientists were able to see a map of all the 20,000 to 25,000 genes in the human body. The DNA sequence was readily available on the Internet.

When the National Library of Medicine in Australia went online, physician Barry Marshall began to research his hypothesis that stomach ulcers were caused by bacteria, not stress. "I found very widespread, dispersed references to things in the stomach, which seemed to be related to the bacteria, going back nearly 100 years,"[8] Marshall said.

Without a computer, he estimates he may have spent 20 years collating data without ever seeing a connection. Instead—to the relief of everyone infected with *Helicobacter pylori (H. pylori)*—he was able to complete his research and prove his theory in only a few years.

Although he had been laughed off the stage by the medical community when he first presented his ideas, Marshall won the 2005 Nobel

Prize in Medicine. His insight into ulcers ultimately saved 500,000 lives a year and rendered a multibillion-dollar drug market obsolete.[9] (Astonishingly enough, the new treatment for peptic ulcers turned out to be antibiotics, not Valium.) By proving that diseases could be infectious in origin, using evidence that was impossible to ignore, Marshall made a discovery that had huge implications for medicine in general. A paradigm shift was beginning to take place.

BREAKTHROUGHS IN PAIN

A pioneer in recognizing the need for a more compassionate and humanistic approach to medicine, Norm Shealy, MD, created a physician's organization in 1978 to bring together the leaders in the emerging area of holistic medicine. As a Harvard-trained neurosurgeon, Dr. Shealy had originally viewed pain as a nervous system disorder. When he saw that our existing medical knowledge had left us without enough treatments for pain, he looked for ways to get the brain to ignore the messages from the pain receptors. This led to his groundbreaking work in the development of two of the most widely used treatments for pain: dorsal column stimulation and transcutaneous electrical nerve stimulation (TENS).

In the early 1970s, Dr. Shealy created one of the country's first comprehensive pain rehabilitation programs in La Crosse, Wisconsin. It was the only program in the country to take a holistic approach to treating pain. Infused with his intelligence, creativity, and insatiable curiosity, the center also became an incredible laboratory for introducing some of the most innovative and successful approaches to treating chronic pain. In Dr. Shealy I found a mentor and was introduced to a model of health care that has influenced my entire career in medicine.

In order to increase his ability to research and experiment with options for treating pain, Dr. Shealy brought together the thought leaders in mind-body medicine, nutrition and herbal medicine, homeopathic medicine, and acupuncture, who were pioneering a new medicine, one that healed the whole person—not just the body, but also the mind and spirit. He called the group the American Holistic Medical Association

(AHMA). It was designed around an open-minded approach that integrated mainstream medicine with evidence-based alternatives.

AN UNEXPECTED BLOW TO MAINSTREAM MEDICINE

At the NIH, surprising developments were beginning to take place. It was obvious that more and more people were using alternative therapies, but doctors did not know exactly how commonplace it was for Americans to seek help outside of conventional medicine.

In 1993, David Eisenberg, MD, and his colleagues published their findings about the prevalence, costs, and uses of unconventional medicine in the *New England Journal of Medicine*.[10] The results shook the mainstream medical community to the core. Not only were Americans seeing alternative therapy practitioners; they were seeing them more often than their primary care physicians![11] Worse for mainstream medicine, patients were spending almost a billion dollars more on unconventional therapies than on hospitalizations by conventional physicians.[12]

Patients were seeking alternative treatment for conditions as varied as arthritis, chronic back pain, renal failure, eating disorders, and cancer.[13] The Food and Drug Administration reported that Americans were receiving 9 million to 12 million alternative treatments every year from acupuncture alone.[14]

Dr. Eisenberg also revealed that the majority of patients (83 percent) had initially sought conventional treatment for their conditions, but when they turned to alternative therapies, most (72 percent) did not mention it to their primary care physicians.[15]

As a result, doctors were taken completely by surprise. We had assumed that conventional medicine had the corner on the market in health care. This new information told us: "Wake up! Your patients are not getting better. They're having to look elsewhere." It let us know we'd dropped the ball and lost touch with our patients.

That few patients were mentioning their efforts to find alternative solutions, Dr. Eisenberg suggested, may have been because physicians lacked adequate knowledge of alternative techniques. He and his colleagues recommended that medical schools begin to include information about these therapies in their curricula so they could be of better service to their patients.[16]

Not long afterward, the government allocated $1 million to create a division of the National Institutes of Health devoted to the study of complementary and alternative medicines. The NIH had never before been open to considering alternative treatments.

It was an unprecedented opportunity for the alternative medical community to bring the kind of rigorous research we needed to test the unconventional techniques that seemed to be working with our patients. If we did not hold alternative treatments to the same standards as conventional medicine, we would never persuade mainstream doctors that alternative approaches could help their patients.

More important, we had to learn how to bring this rigorous evaluation to our studies so we, too, could separate treatments that were genuinely effective from those that were only wishful thinking.

All along, conventional medicine has been vulnerable to the powerful cadre of pharmaceutical companies and impressive research labs that sometimes promote drugs after blatantly inadequate studies. Alternative medicine has often fallen prey to promising treatments that have no more support than folklore, unquestioned ancient traditions, or sleight of hand by charismatic practitioners.

Now that those of us in the integrative health care community had managed to start a conversation about alternative techniques, the last thing we wanted to see was slipshod studies that wouldn't be taken seriously. We had long conversations with the medical science research faculties at the major universities funded by the NIH, who had been doing excellent research for years. We were determined to learn as much as possible about how to do these studies. It was essential that the research get both the scientific method and the alternative treatment right. If either one failed, the studies would be moot.

At the time, it was hard to find studies that got both of these things right. Most in the alternative medical community were clinicians seeing patients, not researchers trained in a scientific methodology that could meet the standards of the NIH.

Now that there was prospective funding for research into alternative methodologies, we were ultimately going to need to train clinicians to attain a higher standard of research and to interest trained researchers in studying alternative techniques. For the first time, my colleagues and I saw an opening, a chance to provide verifiable evidence of some of the things we had seen work in clinical practice.

We seized the moment.

GETTING ACUPUNCTURE APPROVED BY THE NIH

As president of the American Academy of Medical Acupuncture, Joe Helms contacted the NIH to ask about the process. In response, the NIH flew a group of scientists to Arizona to meet with 25 of us from the AAMA and the AAMA's research foundation.

The representatives of NIH explained to us in great detail exactly what kind of evidence we would need to provide. They described the kind of studies they would consider viable and pointed out the importance of following precise protocols to avoid the invalidation of our results. The NIH held a high standard for medical evidence, and we would need to reach it in order to meet the burden of proof if we wanted our studies to be reviewed at an NIH technology assessment conference.

During that meeting, we outlined the designs for three research projects that showed the greatest promise of demonstrating the efficacy of acupuncture. We focused on the treatment of osteoarthritis of the knee, postoperative nausea and vomiting, and low back pain.

Brian Berman, MD, a family physician who had trained in homeopathy in England, took on the osteoarthritis study. Dr. Berman had already received a $1 million matching grant for research into alternative medicine treatments from a British patron and the University of Maryland Medical School. With it, he had created an alternative medicine program in the Department of Anesthesia at the university, which he soon built into the largest NIH-funded center devoted to the study of complementary and alternative medicine. Much of his initial research efforts were focused on acupuncture for knee osteoarthritis.

Dr. Berman and I had trained together in acupuncture in Dr. Helms's program at UCLA. For several years, I served on Berman's external scientific advisory board and acted as chair of the committee for 2 years. His goal, like mine, was to create a body of research that held up to the NIH's scrutiny. The NIH had established the gold standard for research. If we could meet its requirements, acupuncture would be validated as a legitimate medical therapy.

That meant fully complying with the agency's consensus process. Established in 1977, the NIH Consensus Development Program holds major conferences across the country, with the purpose of producing evidence-based consensus statements about new or controversial techniques and devices in medicine.[17]

The consensus process is one of the ways the standard of medical care is established in this country. The panel's findings are published in the *Journal of the American Medical Association* and can make or break any new approach to medical care. After a thorough review of the science and hearing testimony from leading experts in the field, the panel announces its consensus on the topic in a public forum.

My first exposure to the NIH consensus process was in 1995, when Dr. Berman and I, along with 10 other medical experts, were invited to write the consensus panel statement "Integration of Behavioral and Relaxation Approaches into the Treatment of Chronic Pain and Insomnia."

Acupuncture got its shot at the consensus process in 1997. I had the privilege of both serving on the planning committee for the conference and presenting as one of the subject matter experts for the program. When the NIH consensus panel announced its findings, after hearing 2 days of presentations on the state of the research and reviews of the literature, it became the first independent medical panel in the country to endorse the use of acupuncture as a legitimate medical treatment.

It was a historic moment.

Very quickly, I used up several of my allotted 15 minutes of fame. Brad Williams, who was then president of the AAMA, and I, as president of MARF, were deluged with calls from the media. We gave interviews to the *New York Times, Washington Post, Wall Street Journal, Los Angeles Times,* BBC, *Good Morning America,* and almost every major news outlet.

The astonished headlines read: ACUPUNCTURE WORKS!

Almost overnight, acupuncture was cool. Everyone wanted to know about it. On television documentaries, acupuncture was sometimes portrayed as an arcane practice on the far side of the world, performed in tiny rooms with strange calligraphy, where foreign patients had submitted their backs to dozens of long, spindly needles that tugged alarmingly at the skin. It could not have seemed more alien.

With the imprimatur of the NIH, the bastion of conventional medicine, acupuncture got a makeover. Here were American doctors in American hospitals subjecting these "new" techniques to rigorous scientific scrutiny and proving it worked. Whether or not they learned to practice it themselves, mainstream American physicians could now recommend acupuncture as a viable option for a number of conditions.

It was an important step. Bringing acupuncture into the mainstream also meant that research money to explore its potential and limitations would soon become available. Not everyone in the conventional medical community was ready to include it in their treatment plans, but this validation by the NIH did create enough of a shift that even the conservative America military now trains its physicians in acupuncture.

At the time, I hoped that introducing acupuncture to the medical community would do even more. With its assumption that the human body is a single, unitary organism, I hoped acupuncture would help create a major shift in the biomedical model in the country and ultimately lead researchers to new insights into how the body works. And it has done that in many ways.

Throughout this time, and to this day, I have served on a number of NIH grant review panels. The grant review process is time-consuming and somewhat arduous, but crucial to assure that only the best studies get funded. It is only through thoughtful, well-executed research that we can move medicine forward. Funding of poor studies can potentially discredit a useful therapeutic intervention. Failure to fund well-designed, innovative, though controversial work impedes scientific progress as well. With limited grant monies available, the task is to identify the best studies with the most bang for the buck.

As a clinician, my goal is to encourage solid research into the alternative therapies that many of us are using successfully in our clinical practices. If we could move steadily in that direction, maybe we could create a convergence that has never been seen before—one that would open the door to a truly integrative medicine.

Discussing that possibility in 2003 at the founding meeting of the Consortium of Academic Health Centers for Integrative Medicine, I was struck by a comment made by Andrew Weil, MD, one of our country's foremost integrative health experts. As I recall, he said, "The objective of this consortium is to eliminate itself, to be so successful that complementary and alternative therapies become a part of all aspects of medicine. If in 10 years, all we've done is create new departments of integrative medicine, we will have failed."

That same year, I was asked to serve as one of the principal investigators on the $1.7 million NIH grant designated to integrate training in complementary and alternative medicine into the medical curriculum at Georgetown University School of Medicine. Georgetown was one of the first medical schools in the nation to receive such a grant. The grant not only made Georgetown a leader in transforming medical education, but also resulted in the creation of a special master's program in integrative medicine, training future policy makers and medical educators, as well as future physicians. It was the first complementary and alternative medicines–oriented, science-based graduate program in the country.

From the very beginning of my career, I have been given extraordinary opportunities. I'm fortunate enough to be in the first generation of physicians in which integrative medicine began to form and mature. Organizations such as the AHMA and AAMA were a part of that. They gave me access to brilliant creative thinkers in medicine, who were always pushing the edge, trying to discover better ways to heal people.

I have two hopes for this book. First, I hope it will help people who are now suffering find a path to total recovery. Second, I hope it will, in some small way, repay the massive debt I owe to those who have trained and mentored me throughout my career. In my understanding, the best way to pay back the wonderful benefit of their guidance is to take up the torch and carry it even further.

Part I
Asking New Questions

Chapter 1

THE ONE-TWO PUNCH

WHAT IF ASSAULTS ARE CUMULATIVE?

Study the art of science. . . . Learn how to see. Realize that everything connects to everything else.

Leonardo da Vinci

This was the moment he lived for. Perched on a single snowy peak surrounded by a formidable range of peaks yet to be conquered, Billy surrendered to gravity. Leaning forward, he slid quickly down the slope, faster and faster, casting plumes of powder in his wake.

With so little effort—less than a thought—Billy was back where he belonged, carving up the mountain with carefree pirouettes, deep into the powerful compulsion that he and his snowboarding tribe called shreddin' the gnar.

Like most 14-year-old snowboarders, he was still considered a "grommet," but Billy Kass could hold his own. His parents had given him his first Never Summer board when he was 5 and his brother, Travis, was 8. Like some kind of rite of initiation, Travis introduced Billy to the secrets of the mountain. Nodding for Billy to follow, Travis had shown him how to ride a slow S-curve to the bottom. He'd been following Travis ever since.

The 3-year lead Travis had over Billy gave him a distinct advantage. At 16, Travis was all flash and fury. Billy was more wry and understated—not that he couldn't have been the one making noise, but that riff was already taken. So Billy played counterpoint.

Gliding down the slopes together, they wove in and out like a perfectly syncopated song. Travis would line up a 180 "fakie," a 360, a 180, and Billy would intuitively echo the moves.

Gillian, the boys' mom, had almost gone pro back in the day, and their dad, David, had managed to build a meaningful career in environmental science that kept him on the mountain and made skiing a constant part of his life. Travis and Billy dreamed of one day making their fortune together with an environmental tech start-up.

At 14, Billy was more of an idea guy than Travis. As he swooped down the mountain, Billy realized that, of the two of them, he would probably be the one to come up with the brilliant tech idea they needed. He decided to mention that to Travis when they reached the lodge. The idea might not come to him for years, but there was no reason he couldn't start lording it over Travis now.

First, he wanted to "jib" the 20-foot rail up ahead with an enticing 10-foot drop to flat. Leaping on the rail, he rode it all the way down, planning a smooth 180 at the end, but he didn't quite make the full revolution. His hand slammed into the rail on the way down and he landed hard, twisting his back and almost wrenching his knee from its socket.

INEXPLICABLE PAIN

The emergency medical team at the ski resort stabilized Billy's broken wrist and sent him to the hospital. Doctors there confirmed that he did not have a concussion and set his wrist. His left knee was very swollen and tender to the touch. If he tried to stand, his knee wobbled so badly he nearly fell.

When the orthopedic surgeon ran an MRI, it showed an anterior cruciate ligament (ACL) tear. The ACL is one of the four major ligaments in the knee. It emerges from inside the femur itself. An ACL tear is a common injury in athletes, and the ligament is so vital to the stability of the joint that it has to be repaired as soon as possible.

The surgeon scheduled surgery for a month later. In the meantime, Billy would have to keep his knee immobilized in a brace. He couldn't even use crutches. When the doctor rolled out the wheelchair, Billy's heart sank.

Travis reminded him that sports injuries were a drag but only temporary. Still, Billy counted the days till he could take off the brace and get back on the slopes. By spring, he would be back to normal again. Or so they said.

After surgery, Billy had to wear the knee brace for another month. On top of physical therapy, he spent an hour every day locked into a continuous passive motion device to keep the knee moving in a controlled way and help it regain its full range of motion.

The physical therapist explained that his knee would gradually become more flexible as it healed, but that isn't what happened at all. As the weeks went by, the swelling in Billy's knee continued. The slightest pressure caused an unusually painful reaction.

Eight months after surgery, Billy was only one wrong move away from full-body pain at any time. Horsing around with his friends in the living room one day, he bumped into the doorjamb with his shoulder. A jolt of pain shot through his arm with startling intensity. After that, Billy had what his doctors described as generalized pain—his whole body ached all the time.

In almost imperceptible increments, he gradually started to move like his elderly grandmother, feeling fragile, afraid of being hurt. Travis tried to tease him out of it, but Billy's discouragement was too deep. He lost all interest in hanging out with friends.

Despite his family's concern, he was sliding down a precipitous slope into depression. Travis couldn't even interest him in daydreaming about their future in environmental tech. If snowboarding wasn't going to be a part of that life, Billy wasn't interested. Under the assault of the constant pain, Billy reeled and couldn't catch his balance, just as he couldn't save himself in the fall. Increasingly, he was in danger of letting that fall become a metaphor for his life. Looking on, David and Gillian were heartbroken to realize that if something didn't change, their son's life was going to be defined by perpetual pain.

During the next 6 months, he would be rushed from one hospital to another. Again and again, the x-rays, CT scans, and other testing would show no pathology. A spinal tap failed to provide answers.

Neurologists, pediatricians, physical therapists, pain specialists, knee specialists—any specialists they could find—were consulted, to no avail. Not knowing what else to do, the doctors would hospitalize Billy on intravenous morphine until the crisis gradually subsided; then a few months later, the pain would flare up again.

When no physical explanation could be found, the psychiatrists were called in. It was easy to assume that if the doctor couldn't find the problem, the patient must be imagining things.

Accusing any patient of exaggerating pain to get attention would have been humiliating. When the patient was a happy, dedicated teenage athlete with a tight-knit social circle, it bordered on malpractice. After a 5-minute interview, one psychiatrist jumped to the conclusion that Billy was "malingering" to get attention and all but told him to snap out of it and "man up!"

From Gillian's point of view, it should have been obvious to anyone—especially a professional—that Billy simply didn't have the temperament of a malingerer desperately feigning an illness to get attention. He had plenty of attention. What he needed was to get back on his board.

Travis was 18 now, heading for the slopes with their friends every weekend, which didn't make it any easier. Even in the off-season, he finagled a coveted job at Oregon's Timberline Lodge, the only ski resort in the country with lift-accessible snow all summer long.

In near constant communication on Twitter and IM, Travis tried to lure Billy back into the game, raving about 20-foot elbow rails, big wall rides, pole jams, jibs, and jumps. He never really came out and said he didn't believe that Billy was in pain, but his relentless enthusiasm was laden with expectation. Whether he meant it or not, it sounded like he felt that if Billy really wanted to, he could shake off the pain.

"Remember that crash of mine where I plowed into that mogul 2 years ago and broke my wrist in three places?" Gillian overheard him saying one day. "Hurt like hell . . . "

"But you went back out with a cast on. Yeah, I know," Billy muttered. The implication did not slip past him; it slid right through, like a sliver in his heart. "It's different for me, Trav." What else could he say?

As the pain became chronic, the growing list of emergency hospitalizations with normal test results started to work against Billy. Rather than wondering if something had been missed, doctors would assume the pain was psychological before they even met him. On top of Billy's chronic pain, the doctors—and an increasing number of his friends—were adding a new barrier for him to contend with: disbelief.

Months went by without any sign of hope. Then one night, David and Gillian attended a dinner party with David's colleagues in the environmental sciences. The keynote speaker was a medical doctor and avid skier. After dinner, the conversation turned easily to their mutual passion. When Gillian mentioned Billy's unusual symptoms, the doctor asked a few questions, then frowned thoughtfully.

"We haven't heard anything that remotely explains what he's going through," David said.

"Have you heard about reflex sympathetic dystrophy?" the doctor asked.

When David and Gillian got home and looked up the condition late that night, they were startled by how well the diagnosis fit.

AN UNSOLVED MYSTERY

Reflex sympathetic dystrophy (RSD) is characterized by severe and continual pain out of proportion to the original injury. It later became known as complex regional pain syndrome.

Widespread physical pain can be caused by a number of conditions. Under any circumstances, it is difficult to make a firm diagnosis. Even when the diagnosis is accurate, the pain's origin is often mysterious. A punctured finger, a bumped head, a broken toe—small injuries usually start the process. The initial wound heals, but for some reason, the pain spreads and intensifies.

When they first heard the diagnosis, Billy and his parents were relieved. Until then, his symptoms hadn't made any sense. After the ACL surgery, he should have felt *better,* not worse. Naming his condition gave it a kind of validity. It meant he wasn't imagining things. Other people had it, too.

"At least now we know what it is," Gillian sighed.

What she didn't realize was that naming a thing is not at all the same as knowing what it is. The truth is, we've known about reflex sympathetic dystrophy for more than 160 years and we still don't know what causes it.

The first doctor to describe it was Silas Weir Mitchell. In the 1860s, at the height of the American Civil War, he spent his days in triage for soldiers dragged from the battlefield with brutal gunshot wounds and bayonet injuries. At 30 yards, a musket ball could pass all the way through a soldier. The damage was almost always fatal. Often the less serious wounds were so contaminated by mud or bits of cloth and gunpowder residue from the barrel of enemy muskets that, by the time Mitchell saw them, his patients were already septic.[1]

What puzzled him more were the men who experienced debilitating pain even after their wounds had healed. A relentless burning sensation around the wound would move to an uninjured part of their bodies for no apparent reason. Gradually, all of their skin would become so sensitive that the slightest touch or vibration would cause them searing pain.

Dr. Mitchell, who would one day be known as the "father of neurology," originally called the condition causalgia, building the word from the Greek *kausis* (burning) and *algos* (pain).[2] "Of the special cause which provokes it," he wrote, "we know nothing, except that it [is] sometimes followed [by] pathological changes from a wounded nerve to unwounded nerves."[3]

Almost 100 years later, physicians were still speculating. In 1952, Victor Kuenkel thought he had found a connection between the condition (known then as reflex sympathetic dystrophy) and the peripheral nerves. He pointed out that when any of the nerves outside the brain or spinal cord suffered injury, the blood vessels naturally constricted and caused pain. But if a patient had RSD, the pain could be prolonged indefinitely. Kuenkel suspected this was because the body had become hypersensitive to the normal levels of adrenalin in the blood.[4] He may have been onto something.

Recent theories have also focused on the connection between RSD and adrenal hormones. Animal studies have shown that these hormones can activate pain pathways after nerve or tissue injuries.[5] There is also some evidence that RSD may trigger and sustain an inflammatory response that prevents the body from healing.[6] But none of these theories tell us why.

It's hard to treat a disease without understanding what causes it. So it should come as no surprise that, according to the Department of Neurosurgery at UCLA Medical Center, the standard medical treatment for RSD "is usually ineffective."[7] Spontaneous remission sometimes occurs, but even the National Institutes of Health admits that people suffering from RSD occasionally experience "unremitting pain and crippling, irreversible changes despite treatment."[8]

Motivated by compassion, neurosurgeons have resorted to radical intervention: severing nerve pathways. Anesthesiologists have administered strong nerve blocks. Neither one is consistently successful.[9] It seems logical that early treatment would help minimize the burgeoning cascade of pain, but there is no clinical evidence of this.[10]

When he was struggling to help wounded soldiers in the Civil War, Dr. Mitchell found that the most effective treatment was amputation. And even that didn't always help.[11] As disturbing as it was to suffer unrelenting pain without an ostensible cause, it was more disturbing to experience the same feelings in a phantom limb.

Since Dr. Mitchell's day, the neurophysiology and treatment of RSD have remained elusive, but the unfortunate progression of the disease has become clear. For the first few months, RSD causes incessant, burning pain with joint aches and muscle spasms. Over the 6 months that follow, it intensifies. Bones turn soft as joints grow stiff. The area of injury, long since healed, remains swollen. The pain is unyielding. Arms or legs contort as muscles atrophy. Eventually these symptoms become entrenched. The patient descends into permanent disability.[12]

To be plagued by such intense suffering—from a trivial injury—with no possibility of relief is a prescription for despair. Is it any wonder that emotional suffering always accompanies this disease? "Under such torments," Dr. Mitchell wrote, "the temper changes, the most amiable grow irritable, the bravest soldier becomes a coward, and the strongest man is scarcely less nervous than the most hysterical girl."[13]

PAIN WITH NO EXPLANATION

The doctors at Cleveland Clinic prescribed aggressive mobilization of Billy's leg in physical therapy every day to treat it. To improve the temperature of his foot and leg, he was given sympathetic nerve root blocks 14 times. Afterward, the relief lasted only 12 hours at most before the pain came screaming back.

In those interludes, Billy could walk, but he couldn't ride his bike or skateboard to school. It was hard for him to cope with being so immobile. Billy had always been restless. When he'd been unfocused and bursting with energy at 10 years old, his pediatrician had put him on Concerta, a drug to quell the symptoms of attention deficit disorder (ADD). It had improved his grades at the time, but this new combination of immobility, restlessness, and constant pain was so demoralizing that his grades began to plummet again.

One of the doctors at Johns Hopkins recommended an experimental program at Children's Hospital of Philadelphia (known as CHOP) for kids under 18 with severe pain disorders.

"We never learned about this in medical school," Dr. Paul Rosen, clinical director at CHOP, explained. "It's pain without a clear explanation."[14]

The intensive physical therapy regimen they used lasted from 1 to 7 weeks and had been shown to be successful in 92 percent of children with RSD.[15] But the treatment itself was daunting. It was designed to push the pain to the limit. Children who were already in intolerable chronic pain were asked to go off all pain medication and submit to activities that intentionally caused them pain.

A boy named Ryan had suffered a minor knee injury when he was 8 and had ended up in a wheelchair with RSD. "Even if the wind would blow on Ryan's knee," his mother said, "he would cry."[16]

At CHOP, the treatment was far worse than the wind: They used abrasives. Dry rice, popcorn, or hard brushes were rubbed against his knee three times a day for about 7 months, despite Ryan's tears. In theory, the aggressive treatment was intended to overwhelm and reset the pain receptors. There was a long list of children waiting for this grueling treatment, even though everyone knew the therapy was experimental. Word of its effectiveness had spread. For some reason, as Robert Frost once wrote, there appeared to be "no way out but through."[17] Even Dr. David Sherry, who ran the program, wasn't sure why it worked.[18]

Time was of the essence for Billy. Everyone agreed that the longer RSD and similar conditions were left untreated, the worse they would get. Already the doctors at CHOP were seeing that treatments that worked so effectively on children didn't work at all on adults. Billy was already 15, so it was important to start sooner than later.

Billy agreed to try it. First, he went off all pain medication, then he started pulling backpacks filled with sharp, heavy objects down the hospital halls. For weeks, he spent his days doing anything that hurt. Some kids in the program couldn't take it and dropped out. With the loving support of his family, Billy hung in there. Even Travis couldn't help admiring Billy's toughness. "I had it all wrong," he admitted. "You're badass!"

By the end of the ordeal, almost all of Billy's pain was gone. It was a huge breakthrough, the first moment of hope after months of pain.

THE LIMITS OF PAIN

Billy suffered from a condition that impairs the lives of millions of people worldwide: chronic pain. In the United States alone, it is estimated that more than 100 million people a year experience chronic pain.[19]

When one of my mentors, Norm Shealy, MD, founded the first comprehensive pain management clinic in the country in 1971, he observed, "The most common symptom in the world is pain, and yet nobody specializes in it."[20] What we did understand at the time was, when it comes to pain, our bodies have a very limited repertoire. There are different magnitudes of pain, but not too much nuance.

If I shine a bright light in your eyes, you feel pain. If I poke you with a stick, you feel pain. If I hurt your feelings, you feel pain. The experience varies, but in very different situations, the response is similar enough that we all recognize it categorically as "pain."

The brain perceives emotional pain more quickly than it does physical pain. If a loved one dies unexpectedly, your nervous system immediately responds. Adrenaline, noradrenaline, and cortisol surge into your bloodstream, binding to your heart receptors, increasing your blood sugar, and priming your muscles for action.[21] The ache you feel in your heart is not a metaphor. It's pain.

With acute pain, it takes a lot more work to get your brain's attention. If you cut your hand with a knife, the cells in your skin are damaged immediately, but before you can feel it, your body has to send out a series of relays to get the message all the way up to your brain. First, your skin cells emit fast-moving chemical messengers—serotonin, histamine, and prostaglandin—to convey the signal to the specialized nerve endings (nociceptors), which quickly pass it on to the spinal cord. The message races up to your brain stem to alert your thalamus and the higher regions of your brain.[22] All of this happens in the time it takes you to say "Ow!"

With chronic pain, the body seems to get stuck in a feedback loop. If you twist your back and damage the cells in your muscles, you may feel pain for a few weeks, until your back heals and the activation of your nociceptors subsides. But next month, when you turn to reach for a doorknob, a jolt of pain streaks up your back. The month after that, you're just sitting in a chair when the pain flares up. Whether you reinjure your back or not, the pain becomes chronic.

While Billy was going from doctor to doctor, searching for a treatment that would quell his pain, we in the medical profession were just beginning to understand that, when chronic pain was present, some kind of complex changes were taking place in the chemical signaling process of the nervous system. Whatever was going on, it was causing chronic pain even when there was no visible tissue damage.[23] That wasn't supposed to happen. Were the chemical signals misfiring? Was chronic pain actually causing changes in brain chemistry?[24] It was mystifying.

As far as we knew, adult brains couldn't change. That was one of the few uncontested facts about the brain in the early 1990s.[25] Pasko Rakic, chairman of the neurobiology department at Yale, had done studies to establish that fact 25 years earlier. Yet, to all appearances, pain became chronic when it moved from the peripheral nervous system to the brain and made functional—and perhaps even structural—changes. How was that possible?

In the pain management community, questions like these were keeping some of us awake at night. I was convinced we must have been missing something. Maybe some of our best presumptions were misleading us. A lot of research was being done in major research facilities around the world, but the data wasn't always making sense. We knew that acute pain arose suddenly, as the result of an injury. Broken bones were set, wounds were stitched; the pain was comprehensible, the treatment was effective.

By contrast, chronic pain was elusive and complex. Aside from its extreme presentations in conditions like RSD, chronic pain often emerged without any particular injury, persisted over time, and failed to respond to standard medical treatments. We had identified many conditions associated with chronic pain, such as arthritis, migraines, diabetes, cancer, sciatica, and fibromyalgia.[26] We had also seen a high frequency of psychiatric conditions associated with chronic pain, such as depression, anxiety, and post-traumatic stress disorder. We had even developed a variety of treatments for them, but the success rate was so limited that both doctors and patients had come to anticipate palliatives, not progress.

The most obvious questions remained unanswered: What did these conditions have in common? What mechanism was at work when acute pain became chronic?

Bottom line, we didn't really understand what chronic pain was. As a result, our definitions were inevitably vague. Trying to encompass all exigencies, the International Association for the Study of Pain (IASP) defined chronic pain as an unpleasant sensation associated with actual—or potential—tissue damage.[27]

Because sensations are subjective, pain was further described as "a perceptual phenomena with a number of contributing factors . . . uniquely experienced by each individual."[28] However true, this was virtually the equivalent of saying, "The world is so full of a number of things."[29] We were grasping at straws.

The trouble was, the old rules didn't seem to apply when it came to chronic pain. Sometimes, the conditions we assumed would not cause chronic pain *did* and the conditions we expected to cause chronic pain *didn't*.

It would not have surprised anyone if patients with osteoarthritis had chronic pain. It was a degenerative condition with visible wear and tear on the joints. So why were only 12 percent of the people with osteoarthritis experiencing pain?[30]

When young boys were sent off to fight a war on foreign soil, many of them spent months in constant fear for their lives. If they suffered from the chronic emotional pain of post-traumatic stress disorder (PTSD) when they returned, it was understandable. So why did only 15 percent of combat veterans develop PTSD?[31]

At the time, we couldn't respond to these questions. Nothing we knew could explain the underlying mechanism of chronic pain.

Ironically, we were surrounded by clues.

WHAT'S SETTING THE FIRES?

All of us in the medical community were seeing patients with increasingly complex symptoms, in addition to chronic pain. Autoimmune disorders and inflammatory conditions were on the rise. Instead of coming in with a simple shoulder pain or stomach flu, patients of all ages were presenting with a variety of complaints at once.

From the beginning of my residency, I had seen patients with a plethora of symptoms. I couldn't help wondering what underlying condition linked them all together. If migraines, fatigue, irritable bowel syndrome, and PMS were all occurring in one person, I suspected there must be a common denominator.

Unfortunately, as Dr. Rosen at CHOP pointed out, medical school hadn't prepared us for this. The standard medical model was based on the motto One Visit, One Problem. Yet in practice, all of us were seeing patients that didn't fit into a single box. Worse, doctors were increasingly beginning to specialize, taking the distinction even further: One Doctor, One Condition.

As Kurt C. Stange, MD, editor of *Annals of Family Medicine,* noted, the "rise in specialization has led to breathtaking advances from isolating, partitioning, and manipulating the components of physical, biological, and human systems," but we have not made comparable advances in our ability to integrate and personalize the data. "As a result, our ability to turn information into knowledge and knowledge into wisdom has diminished."[32]

He continues: "Healing requires relationships—relationships which lead to trust, hope, and a sense of being known. But our healthcare system doesn't deliver healing. It doesn't deliver relationships. Increasingly it delivers commodities that can be sold, bought, quantified, and incentivized. While the whole—whole people, whole systems, whole communities—gets worse."[33]

Shortly after I opened my practice, a patient showed up in my office complaining of insomnia. For years, she had been taking sleeping pills prescribed by another doctor and simply wanted to renew her prescription. When I asked about her health, she said she was also seeing a gynecologist for PMS and a gastroenterologist for irritable bowel syndrome. Each symptom was being treated—by the patient and her doctors—as a completely separate problem, as if her overall health had nothing to do with her condition.

Then, as now, there was no oversight to ensure that all the medications and treatment plans were compatible. Patients were being given the same medications twice. A stomachache that was a side effect of a medication prescribed by a general practitioner could easily be treated by an internist who didn't know the patient was taking that medicine. Realizing the problem, the medical community pushed for electronic medical records, to give them access to the full scope of their patients' treatments. Articles bemoaning the "fragmentation of medicine" began to appear in the major medical journals more regularly. But there was a bigger issue: No one was treating the whole patient.

All around me I saw colleagues adhering to a sophisticated and well-intentioned medical model that didn't seem to be asking the right questions. What we were seeing were layers of increasingly complex conditions, often accompanied by pain that could not be explained by our current level of understanding. Our solution had been to intensify our focus on one thing at a time—a good strategy in some situations, but not when it came to the human body.

I was beginning to wonder whether some of these seemingly unrelated conditions were having a cumulative effect. If my suspicions were correct, we would never be able to discover the connections with a One Doctor, One Condition approach. We had to look beyond that.

It was as if fires were breaking out all over the place. As doctors, we were doing our best to put each of them out but never taking the time to ask: What's setting those fires?

In a unified human organism, how was it possible to imagine the symptoms were unrelated? There had to be a connection. In clinical practice, that certainly seemed to be true. As I worked with patients, it became increasingly obvious to me that whenever we treated one symptom—and not the whole spectrum of symptoms—patients improved, but often, their overall health was still impaired. Many of them would come back later with more complications.

Surely some underlying condition was affecting the whole organism, causing this outbreak of symptoms. If only we knew what it was.

THE NEED TO KNOW

From the beginning of my medical training, I was always fascinated by the concept of healing. Healing is very different from repairing. Great physicians—like so many I have had the privilege of working with—are not mechanics but skilled clinicians who understand that it is not their job to heal, but to facilitate healing.

My first exposure to the concept of healing was as an undergraduate at Dickinson College when I took a meditation training program. Meditation was not exactly a required course for a chemistry major, but why go to college if you can't do some intellectual exploring? Healing the body through the mind was an intriguing idea, and I realized that if I was going to make any sense out of this meditation stuff, I needed to study the brain. In my junior year, I arranged to take an elective in sleep research at the Hershey Medical Center under the supervision of Anthony Kales, MD, one of the leaders in the emerging field of sleep medicine. The elective evolved into what would become my honors thesis on the neurophysiology of sleep. My work involved not just a great deal of study, but also way too many nights in the lab monitoring sleeping cats.

The research left me sleep deprived and my subjects well rested, but it ignited a deep fascination with the neurosciences that is with me to this day. When I applied to medical school, I assumed I would become a neurologist, but the year I spent in Monterey watching internist Hector Prestera, MD, heal hopeless patients with acupuncture had an unforeseen impact. Dr. Prestera was one of the first physicians in the country to incorporate acupuncture into his medical practice. In that year, he introduced me to a completely different perspective. He taught me that health and illness existed on a continuum.

Acupuncture operates on the presumption that illness is a disruption of the flow of the body's energies and provides a systematic way to diagnose the energy flow and correct it. I observed him treat hundreds of patients and saw for myself how powerful and successful acupuncture therapy could be for a multitude of medical conditions.

Once I started medical school, I quickly learned to stop asking whether acupuncture might help some of our patients. Even the most open-minded attending physicians on my rotations considered acupuncture voodoo medicine. There are few ways to make you feel crazier faster than having your esteemed medical professors tell you with absolute authority that "you did not see what you saw" and dismiss your experience as essentially a delusional episode.

Gillian's growing frustration over the insulting way doctors treated Billy was an experience I'd had as a doctor all too often. I had seen the same kind of dismissal myself in medical school any time I mentioned acupuncture. I'd also observed my professors dismissing patients' symptoms because they "didn't make any sense" or "the medication could not possibly cause that side effect." I was mystified by the widespread practice of ignoring evidence. As I understood it, scientists were supposed to investigate.

Acupuncture was dismissed as voodoo because it did not make sense in light of the way we understood the body to work. Yet acupuncture was one of the oldest systems of healing in the world, based on evidence that not even our most elevated institutions could claim: more than 2,500 years of clinical experience. Acupuncture was practiced not only by the Chinese, but it had also been integrated into Western medical systems in France and Germany with excellent outcomes. Beyond that, I had seen it work.

Increasingly I began to see my medical training as indoctrination into a belief system about health and illness rather than the science it claimed to be. We seemed to have reached a point where if we didn't understand the mechanism of how something worked in the body, then the phenomenon didn't exist.

In his book, *Ignorance: How It Drives Science,* Stuart Firestein wrote, "Being a scientist requires having faith in uncertainty, finding pleasure in mystery, and learning to cultivate doubt. There is no surer way to screw up an experiment than to be certain of its outcome."[34]

The genius of the scientific method is that it doesn't settle for an easy answer or a permanent solution. The "facts" are meaningful because they are constantly being examined and refined: "A new observation, a more honest observation, can always alter them."[35]

In my long and enduring medical education, it became obvious to me very early on that the vast majority of medical professionals are not practicing medicine from these scientific principles. It appears that the urge for investigation has been replaced by the comfortable illusion of having all the answers. Too much of the time, it seemed to me that doctors were not asking the right questions, if they were willing to ask any questions at all. Privately I assured myself that when I practiced neurology, I would continue to investigate a variety of alternative methods, as Dr. Prestera did.

In the meantime, my first clinical rotation on the neurology service in medical school exposed me to one interesting neurological case after another. Clinically, a neurologic diagnostic exam was elegant. Subtle observations—the loss of vibratory sensation in an ankle, the nuances of specific memory deficits, the wormlike movement of muscles in the tongue—revealed significant clues about impairments in the brain or peripheral nervous system. With such a highly refined capacity for analysis, I expected the practice of neurology to be even more impressive.

It came as a shock to discover that a sophisticated diagnosis was all we had to offer the majority of our patients. In neurology, it seemed, scientists had learned to identify the problem but had made very little progress toward finding solutions.

One day, we diagnosed a beloved professor, Gordon Zink, with amyotrophic lateral sclerosis (also known as Lou Gehrig's disease, although it turns out that Lou Gehrig may not have had ALS). One of the top osteopathic practitioners in the country, he had been known as "a rapid fire lecturer who ripped through an amazing amount of material in an hour."[36] Richard J. Clofine, DO, one of Dr. Zink's many devoted students, explained that before he died, the voice that had inspired a generation of students had grown weak. He could barely move his arms or legs. It was a struggle for him to talk or even swallow. It was painful to watch such a highly revered practitioner lose his touch and slowly die of a particularly miserable disease.[37]

To me, it was devastating to realize that all we could do was inform him that he had a fatal neurodegenerative disease. Dr. Zink was ultimately seen by some of the most accomplished neuroscientists in the world, yet there was nothing anyone could do to help.

Until that moment, I had been staving off my disillusionment, but this diagnosis made it personal. I couldn't bear the prospect of a lifetime of giving patients devastating diagnoses with no hope. My dream of a career in neuroscience was over. For the next three years, while I finished my medical degree, I agonized over the decision. But as I progressed through my clinical rotations, the limitations of our entire medical system became even more apparent.

Western medicine was outstanding at treating acute trauma and illness, but we still had little insight into the etiology (cause) and treatment of many chronic illnesses. We were frankly abysmal at treating chronic pain. The way we treated the patients suffering with chronic conditions, especially pain, was even worse. It was as if these patients represented unknowns that were an affront to Western medical science. I observed firsthand how quickly—and often, cynically—these patients were dismissed as malingerers or depressives and sent to psychiatrists.

My brief exposure to an alternative philosophy of medicine helped save me from falling into that trap. I knew that not all doctors treated patients as if they were the problem. Some doctors assumed that if they couldn't make sense of the patients' symptoms, they were missing a connection. Whatever medicine I practiced, I knew I had to be that kind of doctor. I was not willing to spend my medical career making elegant diagnoses rather than finding elegant solutions to illness and pain. As a doctor, my priority was to help people get well.

Realizing it was important to have a solid foundation in mainstream medicine, I applied to the Family Medicine Program at Georgetown University Medical School. Family medicine is a medicine of the whole person. Since it puts health and well-being first, it was a better fit for me. But I was still convinced that, if I were going to really help people, I would need a broader range of tools than those of conventional medicine.

For me, cultivating a deep diversity of knowledge was not just an early academic decision. It is my philosophy of life. Then, as now, I believed that the greater my knowledge base, the more effectively and intelligently I could evaluate my patients' conditions, apply any given techniques, and integrate them with others. I was driven by the desire to improve our understanding of the very nature of our health: how we get sick, why we stay sick, and how we can recover.

I was beginning to understand that the best medicine always involved investigation. As far back as 1950, Cambridge professor William I. B. Beveridge had described the approach required for the kind of medicine I would soon devote my life to. "We need to train our powers of observation," Beveridge wrote, "to cultivate that attitude of mind constantly on the look-out for the unexpected and make a habit of examining every clue. . . . The scientist who has an independent mind and is able to judge the evidence on its merits, rather than in light of prevailing conceptions, is the one most likely to be able to realize the potentialities in something really new. He also needs imagination and a good fund of knowledge, to know whether or not his observation is new and to enable him to see the possible implications."[38]

In the 1980s, we called that holistic medicine, then complementary and alternative medicine, integrative medicine, and functional medicine. I prefer to think of it as simply excellent medicine.

MEETING BILLY

When I first saw Billy in the waiting room at my clinic in Arlington, Virginia, he was 18 years old. Slumped into a chair with a cap pulled down over his eyes, he wore earbuds that kept him wrapped in a cocoon, protected from the surrounding sounds that would worsen his pain.

Three years of poking and prodding by medical professionals had taken a toll. Cordial greetings from doctors didn't stir up courtesy in Billy anymore. He was surly and quiet. When one of his parents nudged him to answer my questions, he spoke in monosyllables, never meeting my eyes.

After enduring the CHOP desensitization regime like a trooper, he had been so glad to return to his life that it took awhile to admit he still wasn't feeling 100 percent. The hypersensitivity was gone, but he was increasingly fatigued and had trouble concentrating at school. He had chronic daily headaches, and they were getting worse.

By the time we met, I was one of the few doctors in the country board certified in family medicine, pain medicine, and acupuncture. The medical team at the Kaplan Center included physicians specializing in nonsurgical treatment of chronic pain and illness, licensed physical therapists, a nurse practitioner, a psychotherapist, a registered dietitian, two registered nurses, and a certified massage therapist. As it happened, I had a particular interest in reflex sympathetic dystrophy and had just gotten back from a conference on RSD at Johns Hopkins. It was a unique phenomenon, and pain specialists tended to gravitate toward it like an unsolved mystery. We were all curious about what was causing it and, more important, how to fix it.

With Billy, I started asking questions about his history and wondering how the things he told me could be related. Taken together, how could they have laid the groundwork for RSD in the first place? And why, after he'd improved so much, was he still having headaches?

As a start, I took a very comprehensive history. In my initial 1½-hour intake, I always cast a wide net, listening carefully, getting the whole story, and—most important—believing what the patient tells me. From there, we have access to a wide range of therapeutic possibilities that treat the whole person, not just the separate symptoms. I keep my mind open, looking for the best way to facilitate the body's natural ability to heal.

But the question remained: Why would a healthy adolescent develop such a devastating illness when most kids in his situation would have completely recovered within 6 weeks? *What else was going on?* Billy was just grateful that his pain had been alleviated, yet I couldn't help wondering: *Had we really gotten to the bottom of this?* Something had primed his nervous system and set him up for this horrific condition. Could there be a lingering toxicity in his body, preventing him from fully recovering?

Like his brother, Travis, Billy had been a constant blur of athletic activity. The two boys had spent as much time as possible outdoors on bikes, skateboards, skis, snowboards—whatever they could find. All of that activity had been accompanied by more sprained ankles, twisted knees, and hairline fractures than either of their parents could tally, but they had always healed quickly.

Vigorous athletes themselves, David and Gillian took it for granted that the boys came from sturdy stock. In the last few years, it had been getting harder for Billy to recover. It hadn't been so noticeable that he had become what psychologists call "the identified patient" in the family, but when I pressed for details, the pieces fell into place for Gillian. "Since we moved into this house 5 years ago, Billy has gotten a lot more colds and ear infections than he did at the other place. The doctor ends up prescribing antibiotics three or four times a year. We used to joke that Billy was allergic to the house!"

The house was at least 60 years old. Over the years, it had repeatedly suffered water damage from storms. A few years earlier, the basement had flooded, prompting the family to do a significant renovation. The builders found black mold behind the wallboards. Mold thrives on the cellulose that covers wallboard. In the dark, with plenty of food and moisture leaking in from the storms, the mold was living in ideal conditions. The builders removed the mold, replaced the wallboards, cleared out the air-conditioning ducts, and remediated the area. But if Billy was particularly susceptible to toxic poisoning, he may have been badly affected.

Earlier in the year, one of my associates in the practice, John Reed, had introduced me to a book on biotoxicity. The work was controversial, but some of our colleagues had been seeing promising results. The author of the book, Ritchie Shoemaker, had graduated with honors from Duke University and was a practicing physician in Pocomoke City, Maryland. His publications in medical journals indicated that he may have identified biomarkers for biotoxicity caused by molds and Lyme disease.[39] It was something no one else had yet uncovered.

Doctors rely on biomarkers of all kinds—objective measurements with clearly discernible results. A dry cough and fever, for instance, may be caused by a variety of things. Biomarkers help us narrow down the possibilities and confirm our diagnoses. If we run a blood test, we can observe that the patient's white count is elevated. A culture of the sputum will identify the specific bacteria involved. A chest x-ray will show the infection in the lungs. With these three biomarkers, we have objective proof that the patient has bacterial pneumonia. If 10 physicians see these biomarkers, 10 physicians will conclude the patient has bacterial pneumonia.

Biomarkers give doctors the objective evidence they need. And yet there are no biomarkers for a remarkable range of conditions. Many of the most common medical diagnoses are based on well-informed deductions, not clear biomarkers. Chronic pain, headaches, and depression are all conditions whose diagnosis and treatment are not based on biomarkers.

A limitation of biomarkers is that while they may tell us you have a disease, they do not necessarily tell us the cause of the disease. Blood pressure, for instance, is an extremely important biomarker. A high reading shows that your blood pressure is elevated, but nothing more. Why is it elevated? The elevation could be caused by temporary stress or an acute illness. Elevated blood pressure could be secondary to kidney or thyroid disease. If your blood pressure is consistently too high, and we are unable to identify a specific cause, we say you have essential hypertension. Essential to what, we're not sure, but we do know untreated hypertension is a significant health risk, and we give you medication. The medication is designed to lower blood pressure, without our having identified the underlying problem. If you take the medication and your blood pressure goes down, you and your doctor may be justifiably relieved. But all we really know is that the medication worked on the symptoms. We have not treated the cause.

Biomarkers can provide us with an objective measurement that a disease is present, such as in essential hypertension, without telling us the cause; in other cases, such as bacterial pneumonia, they can help us target our treatment to the specific cause of the disease. A lot of medicine is based on what amounts to circumstantial evidence. So from my view, if someone had found a biomarker for biotoxicity, I wanted to know about it. John Reed and I drove out to southern Maryland to meet with Dr. Shoemaker and discuss the implications of his research.

Toxicity was a condition already widely recognized as a response to toxins such as heavy metals, drugs, pesticides, food additives, and chemotherapy. These toxins cause damage throughout the body but especially to the brain and nervous system. Shoemaker's research showed that there are far more environmental toxins than previously recognized by conventional medicine. He further argued that a huge number of people were suffering with diseases caused by these previously unrecognized toxins. Symptoms in people suffering from environmental toxicity were extremely diverse, including difficulty with focus and concentration, attention deficit disorder, headaches, sleep disturbances, chronic fatigue, muscle pain, bowel disorders, and asthma. All of these, he reported, were potential consequences of exposure to toxins in susceptible individuals.

Shoemaker discovered that a particular genetic marker was often present in people who were unable to process the toxins from mold and insect bites. Understandably, these people are especially vulnerable to building up a toxic overload in their bodies, known as biotoxicity. When Shoemaker started using a panel of blood tests to diagnose biotoxicity, he found evidence that some of the most insidious toxins, such as mold found in water-damaged buildings and insect bites, had been overlooked—with potentially grave consequences.

In most people, the liver is able to break down these and other toxins (from X to Y), so they can pass through the intestines and be excreted from the body. In about 20 percent of the population, however, this elimination process fails. The toxins are absorbed through the lining of the intestines and sequestered in the body, damaging organs, muscles, and nerve tissues.

Shoemaker had found that when his patients had a particular pattern of gene combinations—known as HLA-DR—their livers could not create the enzymes necessary to get rid of toxins. Anyone's body could be overwhelmed by an accumulation of chemicals, bug bites, preservatives, smog, and environmental debris, but if Shoemaker's theory was correct, a person with this combination of genes would not need unusual exposure to reach a crisis.

If Billy had this gene combination, he might have been unable to eliminate the toxins from his body. That could be the reason he was still experiencing headaches, fatigue, and poor concentration. In fact, it might also explain why his body had been vulnerable to RSD.

Biotoxicity was a theory worth exploring. Following Shoemaker's protocols, we tested him for genetic susceptibility and evidence of inflammatory markers for toxins. I explained to Billy and his parents that it was just a working hypothesis. The theory had not been proven, but we had started to see clinical results in some of our patients. I was hoping we could find a treatment that would remove the toxins and allow the body to heal itself.

The truth is, our bodies have phenomenal regenerative capacities. If they didn't, doctors would be out of business, because doctors don't heal people. All of our medications and treatments are designed to clear the way for the immune system to heal the body. The best surgeon can pull the skin together but can't make it heal. The most powerful antibiotic only works if the immune system responds and eliminates the infection. Doctors are catalysts. With our help, the body heals itself. If it can't, we fail.

Our investigations in medicine help uncover more ways to finesse it. The more we understand about how the body works, the more we can see how little we need to do to get the results. Ideally, I don't need to blast a patient with treatment, but by moving things a bit, I can restore the balance and clear the way for the body to heal—and then see what happens.

THE WHOLE BODY SYSTEM

All of the other doctors Billy had seen had used a traditional medical approach to diagnose and treat his RSD. While it was experimental, even the CHOP program was based on the same basic principles. The CHOP program is a radical intervention designed to reset the pain receptors so they become less sensitive, but it does not attempt to identify or treat the cause. Despite its effectiveness, it is still treating symptoms. My training as a doctor of osteopathic medicine allowed me to bring a completely different perspective.

In 1892, Andrew Taylor Still, MD, founded osteopathic medicine in Missouri because he felt accepted medical treatments were often doing more harm than good. In his day, Dr. Still had come to the conclusion that doctors should do more than alleviate symptoms. They should try to uncover the root causes of pathological conditions.[40] The medical training for osteopathy is identical to conventional medical training, with the addition of 300 to 400 hours of manual therapy instruction. The practices, rights, and privileges of a doctor of osteopathy (DO) are identical to those of a medical doctor (MD); however, the professional philosophy is different in profoundly important ways.

Osteopathic medicine sees the body as a living organism with an interactive structure and function. What affects the anatomy of the body affects its physiology. So if one part of the body's function is impaired, a part of the structure may be damaged, too. Underlying this premise is the firm belief that the body has an innate ability to heal itself. Rather than looking for a medication or treatment to eliminate a symptom, osteopathic doctors are taught to look for ways to eliminate any impediments that may prevent the body from healing.[41]

Another great difference in the MD and DO approaches is that osteopathic medicine sees the musculoskeletal system as a unique organ system. Its health and function are considered vital to the health and function of all the other organ systems. In MD programs, the musculoskeletal system is acknowledged for its structural value, but virtually ignored as an organ system in the human body.

Although the ramifications are still being explored, the osteopathic medical perspective also recognizes a mind-body connection. It is assumed that emotional trauma can be held or "stored" in the body. With manipulation techniques and other therapies, osteopathic physicians are taught how to release tensions and blockages in this organ system.

Whenever I interviewed patients, I was constantly stepping back and asking myself: What else could this be? What is the body trying to tell us? And the eternal, nagging question: What is the underlying connection?

The very nature of being human can prevent us from seeing what's right in front of us. In fact, we're designed to miss certain things. Our eyes have a built-in blind spot (*punctum caecum*).[42] We never notice, because our brain interpolates, borrowing images from both eyes to guess at what we can't see. We sit back comfortably in a chair as if it were a solid object, but at the molecular level, it is in constant motion. We simply don't perceive it. We imagine ourselves standing still, when, in fact, we are racing around the sun at 67,000 miles per hour.[43]

Although we do our best to observe things carefully, we can miss the obvious. The classic test for perceptual blindness, popularized by Christopher Chabris and Daniel Simons, has participants watch a basketball game and count how many times the players wearing white pass the ball. Afterward, participants are asked if they noticed the guy in the big, hairy gorilla suit who came onto the court and waved. About 50 percent of the participants in the Invisible Gorilla test never notice the gorilla.[44]

Knowing how vulnerable we are to missing things, it's imperative to listen as acutely as possible to patients, looking for clues in posture, tone of voice, and emotional state—constantly challenging presumptions and looking for connections. As human beings, there's always a chance that the answer is right in front of us, but we can't see it.

WHEN IN DOUBT, VERIFY

By all appearances, Ethan Lawrence was a vital, healthy guy when he came to see me for his annual physical. For years he'd been speeding up and down the trail along the Potomac River, 150 miles a week, on a Cannondale road bike handcrafted from lightweight carbon fiber. His handshake conveyed vigor, but there was something weary in his eyes.

As I began to question him, Ethan said he didn't have any significant complaints. So I probed further, asking for specifics about his experience before, during, and after his cycling training.

"Well, I have been getting a burning sensation in my chest sometimes at the beginning of my rides," he said. "Not a pain exactly, but a sense of not being able to take a full breath." He told me the sensation usually lasted about 45 minutes. "But I never seem to reach the same peak of efficiency I did a year ago," he said.

Ethan had no history of asthma, heart disease, or anything else. When I did a physical exam, his heartbeats were regular and he had no chest pain. In fact, when he'd had a cardiology workup 2 years before—including a stress echo exam—all the results had been normal. A sports nutritionist had recommended that Ethan snack on goji berries and replace his sports drink with coconut juice, but despite his enthusiasm for "superfoods," they hadn't solved the problem.

Ethan's general practitioner had taken his blood pressure and listened to his heart, but only found what he expected to find: a fit, aging athlete. "You're 52," the doctor reminded him. "All this interval training and powering up hills is hard work. You can't expect to bounce back like you did when you were 25. Maybe your body's trying to tell you to slow down."

Ethan didn't think so. He thought something was wrong. And I believed him, but my physical exam didn't reveal anything unusual. His

EKG and blood work were fine. Sitting on an exam table, Ethan appeared to be more physically fit than most 30-year-olds, but it was after training, not sitting, that he felt tired. I wondered what was happening when he was out on a ride.

If there was a problem with his heart, it would explain a lot. I wouldn't normally expect an athlete who trained like Ethan to have heart problems. But what if he did?

I referred him to a cardiologist, who performed a nuclear stress test to determine how well blood flows into the heart during exercise and at rest. The patient runs on a treadmill after being injected with thallium, a radioactive isotope, which settles into the heart muscle; then a scanner is used to determine the distribution of bloodflow in the heart.

To everyone's surprise, the test revealed a large area of ischemia (decreased bloodflow) of the mid-anterior anteroapical wall of Ethan's heart. When the cardiologist ran a catheter into the heart, he discovered a 90 percent lesion (blockage) of the left anterior descending artery (LAD), the largest and most important artery. The condition was so severe that the cardiologist took the precaution of putting in a coronary stent.

When Ethan came back to me for his next physical, he was cycling without any complaints, grateful that we had discovered his condition in time. Despite his apparent fitness the year before, Ethan had been on the brink of a heart attack. From any point of view, he was a very lucky guy.

Since we're all so vulnerable to missing things, our best chance is to listen carefully to our patients for clues. Unfortunately, medical schools can engender a sense of us-against-them superiority that makes doctors quick to presume they are right and the patient is wrong—not just about the diagnoses, but about the symptoms themselves.

The uncomfortable truth is that there is still so much we don't know about the human body and its symptoms. Just because a doctor doesn't know how to cure the patient, relieve the pain, or make sense of the clues, it doesn't mean dismissing the patient is the most logical thing to do. Hypochondriacs and malingerers do exist, but they are vastly outnumbered by patients who are doing their best to convey their symptoms and would frankly rather not be in a doctor's office at all.

In my experience, patients often tell us exactly what we need to know if only we would listen.

DIAGNOSIS

With Billy, when the tests came back, my initial suspicions were confirmed: He did have the HLA-DR gene combinations thought to prevent people from neutralizing and eliminating the toxins with a markedly elevated inflammatory factor, C4a. Could this be contributing to his pain?

My working hypothesis was that this gene combination was preventing him from producing certain enzymes in his liver. Without those enzymes, the toxins in his body were inevitably building up. This heightened toxicity was leaving his central nervous system in a hyperinflammatory state that, in turn, was making him more vulnerable to RSD. All of the grueling effort Billy had endured at CHOP to stop the pain could potentially be undone if we did not eliminate the inflammatory factors that had ignited the problem in the first place.

If my working hypothesis was true, the treatment should be successful. The protocol for biotoxicity is cholestyramine (CSM), a bile acid sequestrant, traditionally used to reduce elevated cholesterol by interfering with the absorption of fats in the intestine.

Years ago, Dr. Shoemaker found that one of his patients, suffering from symptoms after exposure to toxic algae blooms in the Chesapeake, had recovered after he had prescribed cholestyramine for his cholesterol control.[45] Shoemaker was the kind of physician William Beveridge advocated: one with the imagination and fund of knowledge to see the potential in this unexpected observation.[46] Because many of the biotoxins were fat soluble, Shoemaker hypothesized that CSM could also be used to remove toxins.

I prescribed CSM for Billy, along with a series of acupuncture treatments to help address his fatigue and pain. If the lingering toxicity in his body was causing his headaches and inability to concentrate, they should gradually subside.

In the meantime, I also asked him to see the psychotherapist in my office once a week. His behavior made me think that the trauma of losing so much of his life to RSD may have resulted in an adjustment disorder. I assured him that talking to a therapist could have a direct impact on his body's ability to recover. Billy grudgingly agreed to go to therapy, but only on the condition that his parents wouldn't tell Travis about it.

After Billy had been on CSM for a month, his energy was slightly improved, as were the intensity of his headaches, but he still had headaches every day. Prior to my working with him, Billy had tried numerous headache medications, without success. Early on, I prescribed several others that didn't relieve his headaches either. I even resorted to an intravenous migraine medication, DHE-45. It worked better than the others, but only temporarily. It was encouraging that Billy's energy was continuing to improve, but the headaches persisted. Any one of these meds should have been effective. It was strange that none of them was having an effect. I couldn't understand why.

After about 3 months, I decided to try another injection of DHE-45. This time it worked. It was as if someone had turned off a faucet with a constant drip of pain and now it was gone—not simply improved, gone. Billy was enormously relieved, but I was even more mystified. Trying DHE-45 again, when it hadn't helped before, seemed like a long shot. At best, I thought we might be able to combine it with other medications to keep the headaches in check. Why on earth had it worked so successfully this time?

And then I realized . . . In the last 3 months, the cholestyramine had significantly reduced the toxic load in his body. Presumably, as the toxins were eliminated, the inflammatory condition in his brain had subsided as well. Once that happened, he was suddenly responsive to a medication that had had only minimal effect before. If that was true, it could mean inflammation was a significant clue.

How often did pain patients fail to respond to medication as expected because of an undiagnosed state of inflammation? If pain was a symptom of inflammation, we had been looking in the wrong direction all these years. For generations, we had been using nerve blocks, narcotics, even amputation, to try to stop chronic pain. What if we'd been looking at it wrong?

If relatively minor infections and toxins—lingering in the body, nearly dormant—could have a cumulative inflammatory effect, then a patient's history was far more vital than any of us had expected. What other connections would we discover? The possibilities were endless. A lot of things could cause inflammation, not just infections. At the time, I was so astonished I had not yet begun to realize the implications.

In the meantime, Billy had tentatively returned to his life. His enthusiasm for his dreams had returned, and he was starting to think about college. When winter came back around, Travis texted him with a weather report from the slopes. "Time to shred the powder, bro!"

And this time, Billy was up for it. At the top of the slope 3 years later, he had a moment of doubt—not sure what kind of pain awaited him—then he reminded himself he was a true badass, and he dropped off the edge. No 180s, no fakies, no shifties; he just followed a smooth S-curve down. It couldn't have lasted more than 5 seconds, but not one of those seconds was painful.

If the moment brought tears of relief to Billy's eyes, the impenetrable black of his helmet kept the secret. What the rest of the world could see was that, when Travis slid up next to him on his board, they both pumped their fists in the air.

And then we got an unexpected gift. In his first semester at college, Billy ended up in a dorm room that turned out to have an infestation of mold on the ceiling. After 6 months without symptoms, his headaches came roaring back. He felt tired and couldn't concentrate. His parents had him moved to a different dorm, and I prescribed another round of cholestyramine. In 3 weeks, he was back to his old self again. Without any need of drugs for ADD, his ability to focus was normal and his pain was gone.

I was delighted that we had found a simple, reliable way to help Billy. By eliminating the lingering inflammation, we had cleared the way for his body to heal. But his case left me wondering. How could the one-two punch of mold exposure and an ACL tear provoke a catastrophic system failure like RSD?

CHAPTER 2

LISTENING FOR CLUES

WHAT IF PHYSICAL TRAUMAS BUILD UP?

I'm always trying to see a pattern in the forest . . .

Stephen Jay Gould

On a long country road in Delaware, the final rays of sunlight filtered through a forest of white cedar and black gum trees, as Emily Maxwell and her family drove to dinner. Her brother, Barry Austin, was at the wheel of his SUV, with his wife, Susan, beside him. The kids had piled into the back, leaving the middle seats to Emily and her fiancé, Todd.

Emily carefully smoothed the sleeve of her new dress and smiled at him. Todd was reaching over to take her hand when Cody, the family's huge black lab, decided to do a 360-degree turn on the seat between them, batting dog hair all around him with his wagging tail. Laughing, Emily moved forward to make room for Cody as he snuggled in again. She'd left her seat belt off since the restaurant was just around the corner.

Suddenly, things were suspended, surreal. Sounds and explanations had moved beyond her reach. She was floating, yet not floating, suspended in midair . . . Out the front window, bright patches of green flashed by, tumbling over and over . . .

It didn't make sense. Her only thought came slowly: *What's going on?*

Just before she blacked out, she heard a loud thud. Then everything went silent—not because it was quiet, but because she was so far away she couldn't hear. Yet things were moving all around her, very nearby. Something urgent had happened—a crisis—but she couldn't respond. From somewhere in the distance, she thought she heard Todd's voice calling, faintly. "Emily! Emily! Are you all right?"

And then, as if the volume had suddenly been turned up, the noise began—layers upon layers of sirens. The outcry of steel doors, crushed together, creaking loudly as a crew of emergency medical technicians forced them open.

Emily had no thought of opening her eyes. It was beyond her. But she listened closely to the frantic conversations, distorted by the static of walkie-talkies.

Bright lights glared into the SUV, which now lay crumpled with its right side against the ground, as Emily drifted back into darkness, only to be jolted back by the thunderous whirr of helicopters overhead. An airlift. Someone had to go.

More EMTs rushed in, moving things around. Lots of bustle. A vague sense of relief wafted over her. People were being helped. Things were being taken care of. That was good . . . But no one had come for her.

Emily knew she was hurt, but she didn't feel anything. It was hard to form a thought. She was there, but hidden—in the car and her own mind. The passenger seat ahead of her had broken loose when her brother had inexplicably passed out and crashed into a tree. As the car rolled, Susan had stayed strapped tightly to her seat, but Emily had been thrown up to the ceiling, then down to the floor. She had slid so far beneath the loose passenger's seat that she was nearly impossible to see.

After everyone else had been rescued, a medical technician made a final sweep. Catching a glimpse of a strand of blond hair, he crawled back in to check. The EMTs were alarmed when they saw her there, knowing that if she hadn't budged, something may be very wrong. Working together, they lifted the passenger seat away and pulled her out.

Two EMTs quickly moved Emily to a stretcher, then one of them cut the sleeves of her new dress to insert an IV into her arm. The other kept slapping her face to keep her from losing consciousness. They picked up the stretcher and slid it into the ambulance, then slammed the doors shut and patted them hard to signal the driver. To the sound of raging sirens, the ambulance sped off.

An EMT leaned over her to check her IV. Emily passed out again.

EMERGENCY SURGERY

In the emergency room, medical personnel swarmed around her, checking for injuries. Doctors found her pelvis had been fractured in four places, with fragments of bone scattered around inside. The femur in her left leg had been badly crushed. At first, they were concerned that her femoral artery had been severed. Fortunately, it hadn't, but x-rays revealed a deep vertical split down the middle of her femur.

When Emily regained consciousness a few hours later, a surgeon at her bedside explained that she had been very seriously injured in a car crash and they were going to have to operate right away. Emily heard him speaking but didn't interact. Nothing seemed real. She had lapsed into shock.

After the doctor left, she tried to look down at her leg but had trouble sitting up, so she couldn't really see what was going on. Before she passed out again, her last thought was, *At least I can wiggle my toes!*

The surgery took doctors much longer than expected. Emily woke up in agony. She had never felt such pain in her life. To support the split femur, doctors had inserted a rod down the middle of her leg, then wrapped coils around it and stuck pins through the rod at the bottom, attaching the head to her already painfully shattered pelvis.

For weeks, Emily stayed in intensive care on heavy doses of morphine and other narcotics. Even then, the pain was nearly unbearable. Emily's grief over her father's death, just weeks before the accident, had to be put on hold while she marshaled every ounce of inner strength to get through the day.

Physical therapists came to her room every day to get her out of bed and help her walk precariously down the hall. Emily couldn't believe how excruciating a broken leg could be. Laying in bed was painful, but putting any weight on her leg sent sharp pain up through her hip, where metal pins were holding her pelvis together. Balancing was especially difficult because she could no longer move her toes.

Emily was still in terrible pain when the orthopedic surgeons discharged her from the hospital 4 months later. They were pleased by how well she'd recovered. X-rays showed that the bones in her leg and pelvis had healed. Her body had integrated the metal rod for support, and she was finally able to walk with a cane.

When Emily complained that she was still in pain all the time, the surgeons simply extended her prescription for narcotics. They said there was nothing else they could do. From an orthopedic point of view, she was fine.

Hoping there were other solutions, Emily turned to alternative medicine—acupuncture, homeopathic remedies, massage—but no matter what she tried, the pain persisted. She consulted other health care providers, too, but everyone told her, "You need to be patient. It takes a long time to fully recover from an injury like this."

When more months passed and the pain had not diminished, she sought out two surgeons who'd had success treating chronic pain. They did an MRI of her femur and found scarring around the sciatic nerve. This scarring alone would have been enough to cause her excruciating pain.

After struggling to be patient all these months, Emily was glad to finally have a diagnosis doctors could act on. This was the first glimmer of hope she'd had in a long time. Everything had come to a stop during those long, miserable months. Todd, who had only sustained minor injuries in the accident, had stood beside her every step of the way, but they'd had to put their wedding on hold. If the doctors could address this scarring, maybe she would finally recover. Emily could give up these deadening narcotics. She and Todd could start their life together.

But the expressions on the doctors' faces were grim. "If you'd come to us right after surgery," they sighed, "we probably could've helped you. It's too late for us to do anything now. Why did you wait so long?"

DESCENT INTO PAIN AND DEPRESSION

All of her life, Emily had been a cheerful, buoyant person, quick to see the positive side of things. She had so many good memories to look back on. After her first marriage of 30 years ended, she had found the strength to move on. Before too long, at 62 years old, she'd met Todd and fallen happily in love again.

Now she was taking enough narcotics to put a junkie into a coma. And the drugs barely blunted the pain. She had to take antidepressants to keep from crying all the time. Every time she sought help, another set of doctors told her, "There's nothing we can do."

After almost a year of unremitting pain, Emily felt her optimism failing. With no relief to look forward to, it was harder to encourage herself. Before long, she found herself deeply depressed.

Not wanting to stay in that dark place, she worked up the courage to look for help again. This time, she found Gwenn Herman. After being in a traumatic motor vehicle accident herself, Herman had founded a support group for people experiencing chronic pain.

With millions of people suffering from chronic pain without relief, there was no shortage of participants. Her group had quickly grown into a vibrant, nonprofit community called the Pain Connection, offering group therapy, training programs, live audio broadcasts, 24-hour hotlines, and other resources. "Our work aims to improve the quality of life of those suffering from chronic pain, decrease their sense of isolation and alienation, increase their control of their condition and treatment," Herman explained. "There are many barriers to treatment, including lack of effective interventions, untrained health care providers, financial limitations, and stigma. People with pain fall between the cracks of our flawed health care system."[1]

As Emily was discovering, the traditional medical approaches to chronic pain were limited to prescribing pain pills and antidepressants. Through Herman, she learned about the Kaplan Center. We donate office space for some of her group meetings.

MEETING EMILY

When Emily came in, she was struggling to walk with a cane. The tension in her face and shoulders offered evidence that every step was more painful than she liked to admit. In some ways, the orthopedic surgeons had been right: The bone had healed around the rod they'd inserted, the incision to insert the rod had healed, and the shattered bones in her pelvis had healed. But Emily herself was far from healed.

Looking at her body as a whole, I found it obvious that a massive structural change had occurred and Emily's wounded body had been struggling heroically—and failing—to adapt. Her leg had healed, but every part of her body had shifted to accommodate the changes in her leg and pelvis. Now her skeletal system was completely out of kilter. None of it was functioning well. The compensatory pattern was having painful ramifications.

Powerful medications were beating back some of the pain, but they were taking a heavy toll on Emily's ability to think straight, keep her emotions in check, and run her life. The damaged nerves in her leg weren't sending reliable signals to her brain.

As I reviewed her medical records, I could see that she must be living in excruciating pain. I asked her, "On a daily basis, how much pain are you in—on a scale of 1 to 10?"

Not wanting to seem melodramatic, Emily said, "Maybe a 6 or 7."

Looking at her x-rays, I doubted that. I was reminded again that true listening means hearing what a person *isn't* saying. "Oh come on!" I said, chuckling to put her at ease. "Tell me how much pain you're really in."

Emily looked down at her hands. No one had really wanted to hear the answer to that question in so long that it nearly brought tears to her eyes. "You mean, like sometimes I want to kill myself?"

"Yeah," I nodded. "Like that."

It was appalling to see how badly our medical system had let her down. Emily obviously had a complex structural problem. Yet the orthopedic surgeons had examined her and said, "Your leg's okay." Maybe so, but what about the hip attached to the leg? What about her lower back? Wasn't it just common sense to assume that severe damage to the leg would have implications farther up the skeletal system? She was in pain when she walked. That should have been a clue.

Apparently, they didn't think so. They did their thing and walked away, never looking further than their own area of specialty. Their patient was left with significant back and leg pain that she'd never had before the accident. True, her stitches had healed, but she couldn't walk. Rather than investigating further, they increased her meds, burying her symptoms with narcotics, and when she felt discouraged about that, they gave her antidepressants.

It's sad to say that, in doing so, they were providing the current standard of care in the medical profession. There was nothing unusual about their treatment. These orthopedists did exactly what they had been taught to do. No medical review would fault them. No insurance company would deny their payments. Yet it was utterly inadequate. Chronic pain is neurodegenerative. Leaving it alone was almost the worst thing they could have done.

It is vital that we stop and think intelligently about what is causing the pain, rather than just making it go away. Masking her awareness of the pain, without finding the cause, would have eventually resulted in permanent disability. We should be striving to fortify the body, not to override it.

When Emily came into my office, she was well on her way to a lifetime of pain and suffering because of the very standard of care her doctors had provided. They had followed the old rules of conventional medicine, not knowing that the old model was broken. From the moment of her accident, Emily needed a far more comprehensive analysis and treatment than mending a leg and gluing a shattered pelvis back together. When she didn't get it, her body was overwhelmed and things began to spiral.

PAIN MEDS AND NSAIDS

By the time I saw Emily, there were imbalances moving throughout her entire body. She was severely impaired on many levels. Rather than looking for symptoms to squelch, I began to look for patterns of disharmony. Often, with an elegantly complex system like the human body, there is no simple fix. This disharmony can extend throughout all systems of the body and all aspects of an individual's life, emotionally and physically. It represents a breakdown of the whole. So it is natural that its treatment requires a comprehensive, integrated approach. I wanted to know all of the components—everything that was keeping her sick and in pain.

First, it was imperative that we realign her structural system. All of our organs are connected through the musculoskeletal system. Without structural reintegration, nothing in Emily's body would be able to function well. Simultaneously, we needed to address the physiological issues. She was also complaining of constipation, gas, and bloating.

To manage the constant pain, Emily chronically took opioids. Opioids are medications that are used to relieve pain but have a number of other effects on the body besides pain relief. By attaching to specific protein receptors on the surface of cells in the central nervous system, they not only dampen the pain signal but also cause slowing of your heart rate and breathing. Opioids also cause drowsiness and euphoria. Heroin is an opioid. So is codeine. Opioid medications cause significant disturbances in the functioning of the digestive tract, including reduced gastric motility, increased absorption of fluids from the gut, and interference with the normal secretion of digestive enzymes from the gallbladder and pancreas.[2] The consequences of these changes in her gut functioning resulted in impaired nutrient absorption, creating subtle and not-so-subtle nutritional issues.

In addition, the intestinal tract is home to more than a trillion bacteria made up of approximately 1,000 different species. Researchers are just beginning to understand that the composition of the bacteria in our intestines has a profound impact on our immune systems and overall health.[3]

When opioid medications impair the normal motility and function of the gut, they are highly disruptive to the types of bacteria living there. When we tested Emily's stool, we found significant alterations in her gut bacteria, which we could also expect to impact her immune system.

People take nonsteroidal anti-inflammatory drugs (NSAIDs) like breath mints and think nothing of it. Because they are so widely available without a prescription, it's easy to assume they must be relatively safe. In fact, there are more than 32,000 hospitalizations each year as a result of complications from taking NSAIDs and more than 3,200 deaths a year.[4] These are not benign drugs. They can actually cause hypertension, heart disease, kidney damage, and gastrointestinal bleeding, although these complications are relatively infrequent.

It's far more common for NSAIDs to significantly damage the intestinal tract. This is true for the majority of people taking them. Studies show that intestinal inflammation resulting in intestinal permeability occurs in 60 to 80 percent of individuals within 24 hours of taking an NSAID. With long-term use, 50 to 70 percent of people develop chronic intestinal inflammation.[5]

NSAIDs simultaneously reduce pain and prevent healing. The lining of the intestines is repaired and replaced every 3 to 5 days. NSAIDs dangerously interrupt and block that process. Once the intestinal tract has been damaged, free radicals are often produced in quantities too large for the body to process. This causes inflammation and irritation, which exacerbate a leaky gut.[6]

There is a time and place for NSAIDs and narcotic pain medication, but we need to use them as judiciously as possible, respectful of the body's natural ability to heal itself. The reality is, both opioids and NSAIDs create gut permeability problems.

Without containment, the toxins in the intestines literally leak out through the intestinal walls. Nutrients, which are normally taken in through the digestive tract, cannot be assimilated. Under enormous duress, Emily's body was already failing. If she could not get the nutrition her body needed, her chances of healing were profoundly diminished.

I also explained to Emily that chronic use of almost any analgesic—Tylenol, Advil, Motrin—can cause hypersensitization of a number of pain receptors.[7] Ironically, the end result is increased pain. Studies examining the regular use of these over-the-counter medications have shown that episodic migraines can turn into chronic daily headaches as a result of taking NSAIDs 10 to 15 days a month.[8]

As useful as they were in reducing the magnitude of her pain, the narcotic medications also had a direct impact on her sleep. When she was unable to sleep through the night, Emily was given benzodiazepines. It's been shown that taking even as few as 18 sleeping pills a year—benzodiazepines (such as Xanax), non-benzodiazepines (such as

Ambien), barbiturates (such as phenobarbital), or even over-the-counter antihistamines (such as Benadryl)—dramatically shortens people's life spans. Taking three sleeping pills a week (132 a year) is linked to a five times greater risk of death.[9] This may well be because sleeping pills improve the quantity of sleep, but not the quality.

Patients like the fact that benzodiazepines "knock them out," so they can sleep through the night. On the surface, it's easy to assume getting more sleep means sleeping better. But that's not the case. Sleeping longer in a drugged state, without waking up, does not mean patients are getting the restorative sleep they need to live long, healthy lives.

THE PAIN-SLEEP CONNECTION

There is a vital architecture to sleep, with each stage building on the next. The two types of sleep—non-rapid eye movement (NREM) and rapid eye movement (REM)—restore the body in ways that are physiologically very different from each other. NREM sleep takes place in three stages:[10]

Stage 1	Light sleep with alpha waves gradually replaced by theta waves
Stage 2	Onset of sleep with regular breathing and a drop in body temperature
Stages 3/4	Deep sleep in slow delta waves with a drop in blood pressure, increased blood supply to the muscles, tissue growth and repair, and the release of growth hormones[11, 12] (The distinction between Stages 3 and 4 is based on the density of the delta waves.)

REM sleep recurs about every 90 minutes throughout the night, providing energy to the brain and body with the muscles disengaged and the brain actively dreaming.[13]

Getting enough hours of sleep is important, but the quality of the sleep we get is even more critical. Our very lives—not to mention our sanity—depend on our ability to fully experience each of these stages of sleep. Eliminate Stages 3/4 sleep and within a week we will develop generalized muscle pain. Eliminate REM sleep for several days and we will begin to hallucinate, perhaps even become psychotic. Without adequate REM and Stages 3/4 sleep in particular, our minds can't think well. Any new parent is familiar with the experience of stumbling groggily through the day after being up all night with a crying infant.

What most people don't realize is that our perception of pain increases when the quality of our sleep is low, even if we have slept "soundly" for 8 hours. Ironically, the sleeping pills many people rely on do not support the quality of their sleep in the night and may be heightening their experience of pain the next day. And pain pills may be exacerbating the problem by actually making the pain worse.

When people come to me with chronic pain, one of the first things I do is reevaluate their medication. Chronic use of any pain medication—NSAIDs (such as Advil, aspirin, naproxen, diclofenac), opioids (such as codeine, Vicodin, Avinza), or benzodiazepines (such as Valium, Xanax, Ativan)—directly interferes with the body's natural pain control mechanism. Although it blunts pain initially, it makes the pain receptors more vulnerable to pain in the long run, so the solution is shortsighted.

We need to be smarter than this. Rather than knocking people out when they can't sleep or drugging them into oblivion when they're in pain, we need to start thinking about what's happening physiologically. We have other means to address pain that are more respectful of the body's ability to heal itself. In some cases, the medication itself is actually creating the problem. In those cases, I have to take people—kicking and screaming—off their pain meds. It can be a long couple of months before their own normal endorphin system kicks back in. At that point, their own pain receptors are able to lower their pain threshold and, once again, the pain goes away.

Drugs had helped relieve Emily's pain, but they had also left her with sleep disturbance, nutritional absorption issues, immunological stress, and heightened sensitivity to pain—not to mention their emotional impact.

EMOTIONAL IMPACT

An extremely violent car accident would have emotional repercussions for anyone. For Emily, the emotional strain was amplified by the physical trauma to her brain and body; the trauma of the surgeries; the months of heavy narcotics, antidepressants, and NSAIDs; the abrupt dismissal by the doctors she had trusted; and the onslaught of pain so constant that she had learned to pretend it wasn't unbearable, to spare others from the impotence and misery she felt 24 hours a day.

Emily's recovery was going to require psychological reintegration as well. No one could endure so much without being shaken emotionally. It was all the more difficult because it occurred so soon after her father's death, when she was especially vulnerable. It would be up to a psychologist to evaluate, but Emily already showed signs of depression and anxiety, maybe even post-traumatic stress disorder (PTSD).

The number one cause of PTSD in the United States is motor vehicle accidents.[14] As many as 25 to 33 percent of people show signs of PTSD—such as sleep disturbances, heightened anxiety, hypervigilance, nightmares, and avoidant behavior—30 days after an accident. It's so common that 2.5 million to 7 million people in the United States suffer from it. Their risk of substance abuse is five times greater than normal. And well over half of people in car accidents (60 to 66 percent) have chronic pain, just like Emily did.[15]

PTSD made her inclined to reexperience the trauma, both physically and emotionally. It also made her prone to hyperarousal, so she felt jumpy and anxious. When that heightened sensitivity is triggered in PTSD sufferers, they typically defend themselves by going numb emotionally or hiding out in dissociative or avoidant states. In Emily's case, the PTSD made it hard to take when her surgeons walked away, saying she was fine, even though she was still in severe pain.

DIAGNOSIS

With so many stressors and pain generators contributing to Emily's condition, I needed to step back and reevaluate them all before I began treatment. These included:

- Stress of father's death
- Lung scar tissue from smoking

- Sarcoidosis (a chronic lung inflammation)
- Car accident
- Concussion (unconscious for at least 30 minutes)
- Leg and hip fractures
- Reconstructive surgery
- Cervical disc degeneration
- Chronic pain
- Depression and PTSD
- Headaches
- Magnesium deficiency

My job is to bring the full depth and breadth of my experience, along with my knowledge base and that of my team, to helping patients recover. Although I am able to administer many of the same treatments, I deliberately look for experts who can bring even greater skills to the clinic. I evaluate the patients and conceptualize their treatments, while my team members amplify the number of ways we are able to evaluate and treat each case.

Although the mix of experts varies, my current team at the clinic includes a wide variety of specialties. An expert in regenerative medicine uses an innovative therapeutic approach that can reduce and sometimes resolve the pain of peripheral neuropathy. A family physician focuses on women's issues and hormone imbalances. Since so many pain patients suffer from the emotional effects of chronic pain and illness, I have included a therapist who specializes in eye-movement desensitization and reprocessing (EMDR) and cognitive behavioral therapy. We now have three physiotherapists: one with expertise in pelvic floor dysfunction, prostate pain, and coccydynia; another with expertise in soft tissue mobilization; and another who practices craniosacral therapy. All have a deep understanding of the biomechanics of soft tissue injuries and the intimate relationship of the musculoskeletal system with the vital organs. Since nutrition is crucial to total recovery, our nutritionist adds another important voice to our patient care team. In our regular conversations and meetings about each patient, we are able to broaden our perspective enormously.

All of the members of the team met to make sure we understood the implications of the diagnoses and the treatment plan for Emily. It was essential that none of us fell into the trap of seeing her condition as merely "a pain issue," "a digestive issue," "a sleep issue," or "an emotional issue." Our understanding of the connections between these issues might be limited, but one thing we knew was that, when they occurred inside a single human organism, they could not possibly be separate, unrelated states. All of them were part of an integrated whole, a reflection of the overall state of the person's health.

In my clinical practice, the same passion for bringing a better medicine to my patients that led me to pursue so many specialties was giving me a very practical advantage. When I evaluated patients, I continually shifted my perspective between different medical points of view, like turning a crystal over and over while holding it up to the light.

As an osteopath, I was able to envision the integration of the musculoskeletal system with the functioning of the whole body. When that system was damaged, I knew it had ramifications throughout the body and had ways to address them.

As a family physician, I could think about the digestive tract, sleep problems, and psychological implications in ways a pain specialist doesn't typically consider. But my certification as a pain specialist gave me a greater understanding of the pain generators and the physiology of pain. It let me think about pain in a way family doctors aren't trained to think.

As a medical acupuncturist, I added yet another dimension to my thought process. While osteopathy uses the musculoskeletal system to envision the body as a whole, acupuncture views the body in terms of energy flow. My own perspective augmented ancient Eastern insights with cutting-edge Western neurophysiology, based on the latest research in our medical journals.

When I practice acupuncture, I do it with an awareness of the neuroanatomical, neuro-endocrinological, physiological, neurological, and psychological implications. Combining the insights for all of these paradigms allows me to achieve very different results for patients than if

I'd only had training in one of these areas. Seeing the body in such a comprehensive way requires a radical rethink, but I passionately believe that doing so is tantamount to reclaiming the heart and soul of medicine.

A TIME-CONSUMING MEDICINE

Suppose a schoolteacher tells her doctor she can't sleep through the night. She wakes up every morning at 3:00 a.m. A doctor may simply write a scrip for Sonata to put the patient to sleep. Sonata will eliminate the symptom, but it does not begin to address the problem. The fundamental problem hasn't even been explored.

My goal is to treat the patient, not the symptoms. So when I hear that my patient is waking up at night, I want to know why. Is she waking up because of stress? If so, sleep is not the only area that's affected. A good night's sleep will help her body restore itself, but it will not teach her skills for managing stress. It will not help her relax her shoulders during the day or make lifestyle changes to reduce stress.

I ask a lot of questions, delving deeply into people's stories. What has led to the problem? How have they lost their resilience? What can we do to restore their health as thoroughly as possible?

Treating symptoms has trained patients to think that symptoms are all that matter. ("Just give me a pill.") If we can teach them instead that symptoms are like fire alarms, we can all work together to look for the fire and put it out. Taking a sleeping pill is like yanking the batteries out of the screeching alarm. If that's all we do, in some cases, we're shutting off the irritating warning while the house burns down.

With doctors and patients focused on alleviating symptoms, the ideal of good health is completely disregarded. If patients understood that they had the option of being knocked out by a potentially toxic drug or getting a truly restful night's sleep, they might make different choices.

The truth is, getting to the root of the problem is extremely time-consuming medicine. Not every doctor is willing to do it. The approach is very intimate, but it is a true partnership with the patient. I begin by assuming that patients' intuitions about their bodies are relevant. Who would know their bodies better than they would?

At the clinic, our patients tend to be very bright and experienced with doctors. Almost all of them have seen a lot of physicians about their symptoms before coming to us. They have already been subjected to a lot of tests, medicines, surgeries, and other treatments. We have learned to throw a wide net diagnostically when we are asking questions, realizing that there may well be layers of things contributing to the problem. That's why I do such a comprehensive history. I know that multiple systems will be impacted by every aspect of their health and their lives. Knowing the sequence in which these problems evolved will give us clues to potential environmental, traumatic, or psychological conditions that have contributed to their current state.

We all come into life with certain weaknesses and strengths. We build on or diminish those endowments as we interact with our environments. The nutrition and nurturing we receive or don't receive, the traumas or lack of traumas we experience—all contribute to our growth and evolution. Our personalities, our lifestyles, our health, and our disease patterns emerge from these life experiences. Nothing happens in isolation.

DISEASE IS A PROCESS

With my studies of Eastern medicine and my Western medical knowledge, I'd learned to look not for a cause but for a process.

This combined approach has given me far greater insight into how to help patients than I would have acquired had I become a neurologist. Not only that, but in medical school, I began to realize that I had joined an ongoing conversation about pain where the inquiry was urgent, but many of the most essential questions were still unanswered.

The incredible opportunity I was given, as a newly graduated osteopathic physician, to sit on the board of the American Holistic Medical Association (AHMA) has provided me with the chance to work beside and learn from some of the best medical thinkers in the field: Bernie Siegel, Christiane Northrup, Jim Gordon, Gladys McGarey. Along with Joe Helms at UCLA, they taught me how to practice medicine in a way that reunites the artificial division of mind and body, which conventional Western medicine has almost come to consider a fact.

For centuries, the Chinese have studied the circulation of energy throughout the body. They have a deep understanding of how that subtle force interacts with the organs and other tissues in the body. The entire approach is designed to treat the roots, not the branches. Their knowledge in that regard is quite specific.

They have discerned, for instance, that around 3:00 a.m., there is a reinitiation of the energy circuit in the body. As it completes one cycle and begins another, the energy moves from the liver to the lungs. The most subtle blockages in the body can disrupt that cycle and, for instance, wake up a schoolteacher in the night.

If the body is struggling to metabolize hormones (stress hormones, sex hormones, thyroid hormones), it can be enough to disrupt the cycle. If energy from emotions (frustration, anxiety, worry) is being held in the body, it can keep the energy from moving through the body freely. In any of these cases, the energy of the body is imbalanced in such a way that, when the cycle begins again, there is going to be a problem. Waking up at 3:00 a.m. is not random; it's predictable.

Prescribing a drug to force the body to sleep through the problem is overkill. It is like using a hammer when we should be using something much more refined. We should be treating causes, not symptoms.

Whenever possible, we should respect the influence a small intervention can have. Why do we assault the body when a more subtle solution would do?

INSURANCE AGENDAS

All too often, the reason lies in the medical system itself. The financial reality is that orthopedic surgeons are losing money every minute they are out of the operating room. The time they spend talking to a patient is minimally compensated.

After teaching graduating classes of medical students at Georgetown for almost 30 years, I can vouch for the fact that most aspiring doctors have chosen medicine out of a desire to be of service. They want to help others, and they genuinely care about their patients' health. If their primary motivation was money, there are scores of professions that could have taken them more quickly to that goal with a far less costly education.

Despite their honorable intentions, most of those same students soon end up watching the clock and adjusting their practices to accommodate insurance compensation.

Insurance companies have no qualms about being in it for the money. Although they ostensibly want patients to be in optimal health, they would prefer not to pay for it. Every treatment, every office visit costs them money. In a perfect insurance world, they would be paid premiums without ever having to pay for any medical services themselves. Empty hospitals and empty doctors' offices are best-case scenarios for insurance companies. So they limit everything as much as possible. They discourage long-term comprehensive treatments of any kind. Time is not valued, so doctors do not spend time with their patients.

The unblinking agenda of insurance companies in America is to strive for factory efficiency, narrowing everything down to one thing: a single issue, a single symptom, a single drug. They urge doctors to diagnose and codify the problem, provide an approved treatment, and move on. They want it fixed and done. And unfortunately, this bottom-line mentality, with no reference whatsoever to the health of the patient, has had an insidious effect on the way our doctors practice medicine.

Even if doctors wanted to ask probing questions, to consider other alternatives, to treat the whole patient, the influence of the medical insurance companies is like a riptide, constantly pulling them away from the time-consuming approach of comprehensive patient care. The insurance billing model works against it. The fragmentation of medicine through specialization works against it.

As a result, Western medicine is in danger of resembling the Indian fable of the blind men with the elephant. Each man considers himself an expert on the small part of the elephant he touches, without any idea of what he's missing. Because none of the men communicate with each other or respect each other's perspectives, they never realize how all the pieces connect. In some versions of the fable, they don't even know they're blind.

LEARNING TO LISTEN

With a private clinic like mine, doctors have the ability to opt out of that system. We get to work for patients, not an insurance company. We can create treatment plans based on their needs, not on what the insurance companies will cover.

It comes back to listening. Listening is one of the most important things we do for patients, and that takes time. Only through listening closely to our patients and taking time to do a careful, detailed examination of their physical condition can we come to an understanding of what has influenced their health to this point—what emotional, physical, infectious, or environmental blows they have endured; which ones have they recovered from; and which ones still linger, undermining their health.

When patients come into my office with back pain, I don't ask, "How's your back?" I ask, "How's your life?" At the simplest level, what I do is pay attention to them. They are what's important. I have a lot of specialized information, but I prefer to think of it as a shared exploration with the patient, a partnership.

Life is a struggle for all of us. So when I hear about a patient's pain, I can easily relate. Most of the treatments and therapies I recommend are things I've tried myself. Before I hire a physical therapist for my team, I have them work on me. I want a deeper understanding—a body sense—of what they are like when they work with people. When I give supplements to my patients, they're often things I take as well. If I recommend that someone goes on a fast, I can do it with compassion, because I've done it myself.

The better I can get to know the patient and the treatments, the better I can understand the nuances and sense the connections. We do not always resolve every problem or eliminate every pain, but a personal, comprehensive approach is the best way available to get the results.

No single approach can cure everything. All medical perspectives and techniques have successes, partial successes, and failures. It has always been my belief that integrating different medical traditions will ultimately lead us to a new and better medicine.

Pursuing that belief led me to cultivate as many specialties as possible, then to continually augment that knowledge—pouring over the latest research in medical journals, attending and participating in conferences, investigating promising new tests and treatments. Ultimately, I hired a team of experts to magnify our ability to help patients even more. With all that expertise, the best solution can be the most obvious one. As Freud famously said, "Sometimes a cigar is just a cigar."

For a few weeks every winter, my colleagues and I spend alternate weeks offering medical aid to the people of Honduras. One year, Jeff Erickson, MD, one of the group leaders, came down with a bad case of bronchitis. After hearing him cough, I suggested that he take an antibiotic.

Jeff tried to laugh and ended up coughing. "I thought you believed in herbs and spices!"

"I do," I told him. "And the herb-and-spice you need is Zithromax."

LOOKING FOR CONNECTIONS

Treating chronic pain is never as straightforward as treating a bacterial infection. It requires a close evaluation of the setups, compensations, and consequences. A lot of pain generators have been triggered as a direct result of trauma to the musculoskeletal system, peripheral nerves, or the brain. Others have evolved from compensatory patterns that the body has developed to work around injuries, so it can continue to function. All of these generators modify the function of the central nervous system. Sometimes the process starts at the top, in the brain itself, sometimes in the periphery, but all of the pain generators result in neuroinflammation and, ultimately, neurodegeneration.

In Billy's case, the mold exposure had poisoned his central nervous system. The result was excessive, chronic pain. Although I suspected that, somehow, each of the assaults and injuries had built up in his body—preventing healing and cascading into RSD—I had not yet found the underlying mechanism that would tell me how that could be happening.

For Emily, the pain began with a physical trauma. Both her leg and pelvis were shattered. She had nerve damage in her leg and a concussive brain injury. The compensation throughout her musculoskeletal system was her body's attempt to alleviate the pressure, but it compounded the problem. Inflammation across the peripheral nerves and scarring along the sciatica stoked the pain even more. What if physical trauma could build up in the body, too, emerging into a condition that was *much worse* than its component parts?

Even if I could not yet identify the underlying connection between so many overlapping systems, comprehensive treatment was literally the only viable approach.

"You're right to think not enough has been done for you," I told Emily. "There is so much more we can do to restore your quality of life. If we use an aggressive integrative approach, with both conventional and alternative treatments, we will literally take the pain out of your body a layer at a time."

Emily looked as if she wanted to believe me, but her experiences hadn't given her much reason for hope. Listening from the side of the room, Todd was frankly skeptical. He had seen conventional medical doctors repeatedly let Emily down, but as far as he knew, "alternative practitioners" were unqualified pretenders. Any success they had with their bogus procedures was most likely a placebo reaction. It was not much better than hocus-pocus.

If the best orthopedic surgeons had not been able to help her, Todd couldn't see any reason why I would be able to help. But I had caught his interest by listening carefully to Emily and recommending a comprehensive approach. This was the first time he had heard anyone do that.

"Will you ever be 100 percent back to normal? No. Your injuries are too severe," I explained. "But you will be much more active and engaged. That feeling of hopelessness and powerlessness will be gone.

"Can we can decrease your pain medications, be smarter about which medications you need, and put you on much more solid ground structurally?

Yes, absolutely. Can we reduce your pain? Yes. Absolutely. Can we relieve your PTSD and depression? Absolutely.

"More than one thing is going wrong for you right now. We need to address all of them comprehensively. If we treat you, the whole patient, instead of treating each symptom as a separate thing, the synergy will make a dramatic difference."

"How can you do all that at once?" Emily asked.

"We need a team."

For Emily's structural issues and the disc degeneration in her spine, I would treat her with manual manipulation. Acupuncture would relieve her pain and help reintegrate all of her body's systems. The physical therapist would work to improve Emily's flexibility, range of motion, and structural integration. The trauma and long-term physical and psychological stress had impacted her brain's ability to regulate her hormones. She was having hot flashes and sleep disturbances. The physician specializing in hormonal conditions would test and treat her for that.

We would also be using prolotherapy, an orthopedic procedure designed to stimulate the body's natural healing process to repair the joints and ligaments that had been traumatized by the accident and surgeries. Prolotherapy involves the injection of a mild irritant into the tendons or ligaments. A 15 percent dextrose (sugar) solution is most commonly used. This creates a mild inflammatory response that encourages the growth of new supporting tissues that strengthen a weakened structure like Emily had. The principle has been applied since the days of the early Roman Empire in 500 BC to restore stability and flexibility.[16]

Our cognitive therapist would work with Emily using EMDR, a psychotherapy treatment designed to alleviate distress associated with traumatic memories by using physical cues, such as hand tapping and other sounds or movements. In conjunction with talk therapy, EMDR has been shown to help reduce PTSD much more rapidly and successfully than talk therapy alone.[17] Without treatment, most people recover from a car accident in 12 months or less, but some people, like Emily, suffer in the throes of PTSD much longer.

In the year since her injury, Emily had gained 25 pounds and had been unable to lose it, so we needed to evaluate her nutritional status. Testing revealed evidence of abnormalities in her intestinal permeability. The testing requires the patient to drink a solution containing two sugars, lactulose and mannitol. The patient's urine is then analyzed to see whether or not the sugars have been absorbed correctly.

As digested food passes through the long intestinal cavity, nutrients are absorbed through the lining into the body. The intestinal lining provides a barrier composed of many layers. It is designed to allow water and small molecules of nutrients to pass through and nourish the body.

Between the cells of the lining of the small intestine are highly complex channels known as the tight junctions. They act as gatekeepers, selecting which molecules can pass into the body and which should be kept in the intestines. As we are just learning, the capacity of the tight junctures to make those selections is finely tuned by our body chemistry.

When that capacity is disrupted, the tight junctures open too wide and allow larger molecules of digested food to pass through the lining into the bloodstream. The body responds to these molecules as if they were antigens and provokes an immune response.

When that happens, it is colloquially known as leaky gut. In Emily's case, it contributed to the overall inflammation in her body and interfered with the absorption of trace nutrients that she needed to heal. To address this, we eliminated common food allergens such as gluten, milk, and milk products from her diet because they potentially boost inflammation. We also recommended supplements and probiotics to restore the health of her intestinal tract.

"While all of this is going on, all of us who are treating you will meet regularly to discuss your progress," I explained. "We will all be aware of what's being done by the other practitioners at every step of the way. We'll be treating your mind and body as a whole."

Todd smiled. He'd never heard of some of these treatments, but this approach just sounded like common sense.

Emily was ready to try the more comprehensive approach I was suggesting, but before we got started, there was one more thing I needed to ask her: "Do you want to walk without your cane and be pain free?"

WANTING RECOVERY

Very early in my residency, I once went to hear Elisabeth Kübler-Ross, MD, speak. She told an anecdote that I will never forget. As I remember it, she said she saw a patient who had been treated with chemotherapy for leukemia. The treatment had failed. His doctors had sent him to her, so she could help him come to terms with dying.

When she met the man, she asked him to draw a picture of his experience of chemotherapy. She projected the drawing on the screen for those of us in the audience to see. In the center was a nasty, menacing creature, representing the chemotherapy agents. Next to it, the man's meek, mild cancer cells stood by helpless. Beneath the drawing, the man had written: "Thou shalt not kill."

Questioning the man, Kübler-Ross learned that he was a devoted pacifist with a profound revulsion to killing of any kind. Rather than helping the man accept his inevitable death, she helped him reframe his attitude toward chemo. A few weeks later, he produced a drawing that showed he had changed his mind. Kübler-Ross sent him back to his doctors for another round of treatment, and his cancer went into remission, as she'd hoped it would when she saw his drawing. It depicted the chemotherapy agents not as monsters, but as monks, gently escorting the cancer cells out of his body.

The story taught me not to underestimate the power of belief. If a patient does not want to recover, they have the power to prevent it. Once I was seeing patients myself, I made a point to simply ask if they wanted to get well.

Emily, like most chronic pain suffers, found it hard to consider the idea that she might be able to walk without a cane, pain free, but she said she wanted to—without hesitation.

"And now for the bad news," I told her. "Your pain medications are actually making things worse."

I explained that opioids and benzodiazepines create problems, too, but chronic use of almost any analgesic—Tylenol, aspirin, Advil, Motrin—causes the hypersensitization of a number of pain receptors. Ironically, the end result of pain pills is increased pain.

Over the next 3 or 4 months, Emily discovered that, even with the right model, recovery from so many things at once was no walk in the park. Without the pain medication, everything hurt. All of the practitioners on the team explained that the medications had shut down her body's ability to produce its own natural pain relievers, endorphins. Until her own pain relief system kicked in, pain would be her unwelcomed companion. She forced herself to go through the process, keep the appointments, and do what the doctors prescribed, and she had to do it in spite of a constant sense of doubt, suspecting every day that she was wasting her time.

When it was hard to keep going, she drew on the optimism of the staff at my clinic and the patients in the waiting room who told her of their progress. The staff was not suffering like she was, but we'd had the privilege of seeing patient after patient make steady progress back to health. We knew that it would work if she hung in there. For months, all Emily could do was trust in our certainty, because she couldn't feel it herself.

In times when she was feeling the worst, she still recognized that "all of these people were trying to help me. I've never had that kind of support in my whole life. Think about it. When do you have that? It's like having a big, supportive family encouraging you. But you have to be willing to go the distance."

The long-term hope of something better was the only possibility that got her out of bed in the morning. It was the reason she hadn't killed herself, even when she thought it was probably the only thing that would put an end to her pain. As the months wore on and the treatments didn't seem to be making much difference, the idea that it might work was just enough to make her keep trying a little more.

Then one morning, it started to shift . . . at first imperceptibly, then it got stronger. The cloud she'd felt in her body seemed to dissipate. Her thoughts were vivid. Her mood began to change. Todd noticed it without her saying anything. In the weeks and months that followed, her pain diminished, and her body gradually started to grow stronger. Emily didn't know what to make of it, but everything was changing, opening up.

One sunny day in late December, Todd came into the room smiling. "Let's go on a picnic," he said, "and get married!" They got married on New Year's Day.

"I understand now why people say, 'That disaster was the best thing that ever happened to me,'" Emily said later. "It's not that it was good, but that you would never have made these important changes—things would never have been this good—if it hadn't happened. In the end, I'm probably going to be better than I was before the accident!"

Today, Emily estimates she is 70 percent there. She can walk without a cane, but not yet for long periods. When she encourages other patients in my waiting room, she tells them they have to make a commitment, to keep going, even if they don't know whether it's working.

"Because it's an undeniable fact," Emily says. "If I had stopped after 3 or 4 months, I wouldn't be able to walk."

WHAT WE TELL OURSELVES

By bringing so many approaches to bear on her case, we were reworking the neurocircuits to bring them into balance—a place of far greater resilience. Because our team was working with the tissues and structure in Emily's body, all the way through the central nervous system to the vital organs, we were literally changing the body image in the brain. That's why it worked.

It was about listening to the patient, doing thoughtful examinations, running comprehensive tests, then having the tools and the team to address every issue. No one person could do all of this. It's too vast. To make comprehensive changes in a system as profoundly interactive and complex as the human body, it takes a team of experts.

The fact that we were able to help Emily did not negate the critically important efforts of the orthopedic surgeons at all. They had to be there. Before anything else, Emily's leg and pelvis had to be repaired. Despite quitting too soon—shockingly short of a solution—the orthopedists didn't do anything wrong. They just didn't do enough. They had never been trained to think to the next level.

People make up stories all the time about why they're feeling the way they're feeling. There is nothing more human than searching for meaning. Sometimes their assumptions are right, sometimes they're very far off. Those of us in the medical profession do exactly the same thing. We make up a story about why patients are in pain, why patients are suffering.

When patients tell their stories and describe their symptoms to doctors, there is always a lot of information that we simply ignore. We have been taught to look for certain clues and eliminate irrelevant details. We evaluate what we hear, based on what we know. The more we know, the more options we are able to discern.

Once we arrive at a theory, however, it is our obligation to continually test and retest our hypotheses. If our treatments are working, fine. If not, we're missing something. When a young patient's knee heals but the pain increases and spreads, we're missing something. When an older patient's broken bones heal but the pain is so intense she can't walk, we're missing something.

Both of these cases seemed to indicate that, for some reason, the body had the ability to hold on to assaults from the past, even after they'd been treated and long forgotten. Instead of dissipating over time, they appeared to be building up. Whenever that happened, pain became chronic, intense, and inexplicable. Medications were ineffective. New wounds wouldn't heal. An entirely new, potentially devastating condition emerged.

In my clinical practice, we were getting good results by taking a thorough medical history, looking hard for clues, and providing comprehensive treatment. The hope was that, if we could reduce the total burden of infection and trauma, we would give the body enough relief that it could heal itself.

Treating the whole patient was, naturally, far more effective than treating the symptoms. But why were these traumas building up like this? What made the body react as if all these different assaults were cumulative?

I was determined to find the single point of origin.

CHAPTER 3

THE CANARY IN THE COAL MINE

WHAT IF PAIN AND EMOTION ARE SIGNS OF THE SAME THING?

Science is always wrong. It never solves a problem without creating 10 more.

George Bernard Shaw

When he played football in high school, Charlie Murphy was a linebacker. Whatever pain the other team could bring, he was ready for it. After the beating he took on the field, he expected to have aches and pains in his senior year. All his buddies did. "Work hard, play hard" was their motto. And pain was the price.

When he needed knee surgery at 20, Charlie didn't think much of it. Lots of athletes blew out their knees playing sports. Afterward, he bounced back well enough to join the guys for their regular game in the park on Sunday afternoons, but a few months of being tackled on the grass left him hobbling, favoring one leg. Doctors said he'd torn the meniscus in his left leg and needed surgery. It was the first of many.

By the time he was 30, Charlie had gone under the knife seven times: one surgery for his shoulder, six for his knees. After every setback, he took it easy during the recovery period, like the doctors ordered, then went back to training and playing ball, enjoying a healthy, athletic lifestyle.

Coming out of one recovery period, he started doing crunches at the gym when he heard a noise from his spine he'd never heard before. Not good. Still lying on the matt, he froze, afraid to move. *Now what?* he thought. Tears welled up in his eyes.

Frowning, his friend Jerry set down a dumbbell and wiped the sweat from his forehead. "You okay, bud?"

Surprised at the way his own voice trembled, Charlie said, "No, I'm not."

On the way to the emergency room, a deep ache started spreading across Charlie's lower back, then flared up into real discomfort. He shifted uneasily in the passenger seat as Jerry drove. The last thing he wanted was another surgery.

In the ER, the doctor did a quick x-ray, gave him a prescription for pain medication and muscle relaxants, and then referred him to an orthopedist. When the orthopedist examined his MRI and CT scan, he assured Charlie his back was normal. A cortisone injection to reduce the swelling and the pain didn't help.

Before long, he couldn't seem to put his body in any comfortable position—sitting, standing, or lying down. Exhausted from constant pain and lack of sleep, Charlie called my office.

It was 1987. My office had been open for only 2 years. Pain medicine wasn't even a board specialty yet. I was already exploring alternative treatments for intractible pain, but it was Charlie's case that raised the alarm. Charlie was like the canary in the coal mine.

After our heartbreaking failure with Charlie, it was clear to me that our need for a workable understanding of the connections between pain, depression, and illness was not just imperative—it was urgent.

MEETING CHARLIE

At 6 feet tall, 225 pounds, Charlie had an imposing presence. The first time I met him, he was 32 years old. He had recently married and taken a job as a performance consultant at Halliburton. He didn't look like a high school jock anymore, but I could still see the linebacker in his walk.

Scars from the surgeries crisscrossed his knees like hash marks. The surgery on his shoulder had been mostly successful, but it still hurt when he moved in certain ways, and he couldn't sleep on it. Charlie's main complaint was very low back, coccyx pain, extending into his thighs.

The coccyx is literally our tailbone. The small tapered end of our spine is the vestigial remnant of the tail we developed in the womb until we were a little over a month old. We shed the tail before we're born, but if we'd kept it, we'd have much greater balance and mobility. Even without the tail, the coccyx is a locus point for nerves, muscles, tendons, and ligaments in our lower backs. When we're seated, it forms a tripod with our sitz bones and bears most of our weight when we lean back.

Charlie's coccyx may have been bruised or fractured. If they're hit hard enough, the five small, bony segments can be dislocated, but Charlie had been doing crunches at the gym—not something that typically dislocates bones, makes a popping sound, or ignites a chronic coccyx pain (coccydynia). In fact, women are more prone to coccyx injuries than men, because the female pelvis is broader and most exposed.[1]

Strangely enough, my neurologic exam of Charlie showed no sign of nerve damage to his lower back or legs. He had tenderness around the coccyx, but no evidence of swelling or trauma at all. Yet he was in constant pain.

PAIN GENERATORS

Even if my initial exam doesn't reveal the source of the problem, a patient can give me important clues by describing the quality of the pain.

Arthritis in the bones creates a deep ache. When tendons, ligaments, or muscles are damaged, there may be no pain or a dull ache at rest and sudden, stabbing pain with movement.

When the nerves are involved, patients typically describe three very different sensations: allodynia, paresthesia, and/or dysesthesia. With allodynia, things are painful that should not be painful. Gently brushing the skin can cause pain. It's a hallmark of reflex sympathetic dystrophy. Tingling, prickling numbness, as when a limb falls asleep, is called paresthesia. It is not painful, but it can be a sign of nerve damage. Patients describe a loss of sensation, heaviness, or coldness. By contrast, dysesthesia (from the Greek words *dys*, "not normal," and *aesthesis*, "sensation") feels like burning, shooting pain.

Whenever I diagnose someone in pain, the first question I ask myself is: What are the pain generators? Regardless of the situation, it's crucial that we find and treat all of them. When we don't, the others remain active.

Suppose a patient complains of shoulder pain that sounds like arthritis. His doctor takes an x-ray, confirms a slight wear and tear on the bone, and assumes it must be arthritis. Maybe it is. But a lot of things cause shoulder pain. It's very possible that there are also other elements at play. The pain generators may be coming from the tendon, muscle damage, ligament damage, or nerve damage in the neck. We have to address everything causing the pain or we will only get a partial result.

When the patient comes back because his shoulder still hurts, and the doctor puts the blame on him ("You can't expect to feel like you did when you were younger."), it's an easy out, but it's not good medicine.

Unfortunately, the failure to identify all the pain generators is so commonplace that most doctors and patients have grown accustomed to the expectation of feeling better but not well or even back to normal. Patients are grateful for any improvement, and doctors don't know what else to do, so we leave it at that. No one ever seriously thinks that total recovery might be an option.

The fact is, it's not unusual for a single pain to have multiple pain generators. A shoulder injury may involve damaged tendons and/or damaged ligaments and/or muscle strain and/or arthritic degeneration of the bone.

In 1952, Janet Travell, MD, made a groundbreaking discovery about a previously unsuspected way the body generates pain: An injury to the fascia, deep inside the muscles, can radiate pain throughout the entire body for years.[2]

Beneath our skin, the cells of our muscles and bones are surrounded by a strong, flexible bodysuit made up of fascia, tightly packed bundles of collagen fibers with a tensile strength of more than 2,000 pounds.[3] Integrated together, fascia and muscles are referred to as myofascial tissue.

In a healthy state, fascia is soft and stretchy, allowing us to move freely and enjoy full range of motion. Under duress, it can become tight and stiff, creating tension, pain, and diminished circulation throughout our bodies. Overuse of joints or muscles, trauma, infection, or even inactivity can cause it to constrict.[4]

If our skin were stripped off, we'd be cold, but our bodies would still hold together. If we took away all of our fascia, we'd fall apart. The fascia holds all the tissue in our bodies together. But it is not dormant. It is another structural system that communicates with all the systems in our bodies. And when it is damaged, the injury can have wide-ranging effects. Dr. Travell was the first to recognize that the fascia within the muscles can be torqued in ways that cause pain, shorten the muscles, limit their range of motion, and compromise the biomechanical integrity of the system.

Senator John F. Kennedy had turned to her for help in the 1940s with the back injuries that had plagued him since his service in World War II. Despite repeated operations by top surgeons, Kennedy had been left with severe, chronic back pain. Dr. Travell's methods proved so effective that, when he became president, Kennedy took her with him. She was the first woman to be appointed personal physician to an American president and went on to become one of the most important physicians of the 20th century.[5]

Deep inside our muscles, Dr. Travell had found, there are sensitive spots with a long-term memory of previous injuries. A taut band runs through these spots, holding the tension. When the bands are stimulated, there is a twitch response. She called these taut bands trigger points—tiny focal points of muscle tenderness, just a few millimeters wide. Pain from these areas was not related to acute local trauma, inflammation, infection, or degeneration and could not be explained by a neurological exam.[6]

Travell observed that patterns of radiation from myofascial triggers were completely different from the patterns we would expect to see if a nerve response had been triggered. As she began to map those patterns, she was able to confirm the origin of the pain. Studies have since shown that as much as 75 to 95 percent of regional pain is actually myofascial pain.[7]

Biopsies later confirmed that those trigger points are electrically active spindles of muscle buried within ordinary muscle tissue, that are indeed hyper-irritable.[8] In recent years, medical schools have taught the concepts and treatment modalities for myofascial pain syndrome.

Muscle relaxants are sometimes effective. Curiously enough, some antidepressants have also been shown to relax these hyperactive spindles. There are, however, many cases where trigger point therapy is all that is needed to eliminate myofascial pain that has lasted for years.

If a patient comes to an orthopedist with tennis elbow, there is an injury to the extensor tendons in the elbow. An orthopedist will typically inject the tendon with a steroid and call it a day. In many people, that will, in fact, resolve the issue, but in many others, it will not. Frequently this type of injury has also set off trigger points in the extensor muscles. Sometimes there is an additional injury to the elbow ligaments. Unless all the pain generators are addressed, the patient's elbow will likely continue hurting, be slow to recover its strength, and be vulnerable to new injuries, since it has not fully healed.

Direct myofascial release (also known as deep tissue work)[9] applies pressure to the myofascial tissue restrictive barrier until a tissue release occurs. Various forms of pressure are used: pressure from knuckles or elbows to slowly stretch the fascia, dry needling (stimulating the trigger point by sticking a needle into it without injecting anything), spray-and-stretch (a technique where a cold fluid spray is applied to the muscle while stretching it to its normal length), or injecting the trigger with Xylocaine (a local analgesic). Regardless of the approach, this treatment is designed to work slowly through the layers of fascia to the deeper tissues.[10]

The goal is to reintegrate the dysfunctional part into the whole. It is essential to reestablish equilibrium in the system so no one muscle, joint, ligament, or tendon is carrying too much of the load. If an imbalance is sustained, over time, compensatory patterns set in, as the body attempts to bring itself back into balance. Manual therapy and physical therapy can also help restore the reciprocal relationships of the body's overall structure.

DIAGNOSIS

When I checked Charlie for myofascial pain, he had many of the classic signs of taut trigger point bands. Examining him from a myofascial point of view gave me one more layer of analysis to consider.

A few years before I met Charlie, all of us in pain management had read the book Dr. Travell published describing the latest applications of her method.[11] I had also had the unusual opportunity of attending a few of her lectures on myofascial pain. Her work powerfully deepened our understanding of how the body manages trauma and how unwrapping layers of trauma can help the body heal.

My initial diagnosis of Charlie's condition was low back pain as a consequence of myofascial pain. I treated him with trigger point injections of Xylocaine. After four treatments, accompanied by acupuncture and manual therapy, his pain diminished. But inexorably, it returned.

A miserable pattern was taking shape. When nothing worked, Charlie would decide to tough it out on his own for as long as he could. Promotions at Halliburton meant he did a lot of international traveling. When he couldn't take it anymore, he tried doctors in whatever country he was in, desperate to keep his life from sliding off the precipice. Physical therapy, powerful pain medication, nerve blocks—he was willing to try anything. Some of it helped; some of it didn't. As far as Charlie was concerned, he'd even welcome a placebo effect if it gave him relief.

Thinking warmer weather might help, he moved the family to Southern California, but 4 years later, he was back in my office again. His whole life had started to deteriorate. His marriage had always been a source of comfort to him, but now he and his wife were going to couples therapy to see if they could work things out. On top of the back pain, he had frequent headaches. Looking for things we hadn't tried yet, I referred him to a rehabilitation specialist and a neurologist. I didn't care who made him better, as long as his condition improved.

After a few months, the coccyx pain came back. Charlie felt a growing sense of impotent rage. It was completely understandable. With every new treatment, he did exactly what the doctors were telling him to do, but he was still getting worse. Frustrated and frightened, he worried that if the pain kept coming back, he wouldn't be able to focus at work. And what would he do then?

As I listened to Charlie, I felt a sorrowful sense of déjà vu. I was starting to hear this story more and more from the patients who came to me. Chronic daily pain was interfering with their lives. Every time they sought different doctors, they got different assessments, because there was no distinctive etiology of the pain. None of the standard treatments had a significant effect. Ultimately, it was a dead end: lots of doctors, lots of studies, lots of procedures, but no help.

What was going on with these people? Why were our best practices so blatantly ineffective? In Freud's day, mysterious conditions without physical explanations were regarded as hysteria. We knew better now, but that didn't mean we had an explanation.

I recommended that Charlie try Elavil, a tricyclic antidepressant (TCA). Studies had shown it could be useful for headaches and certain pain conditions. When we combined it with regular sessions of acupuncture and manual therapy, we were able to manage his pain. Charlie could then put more energy into his marriage, engage in an active social life, go back to working out, and devote himself to the work he loved. He was extremely high functioning, as long as he could minimize the pain with our treatment plan. It wasn't a solution, but it was better than the constant suffering he'd been going through.

Then, in 1990, things heated up at work. During the Gulf War, Charlie was working stressful 14-hour days through the weekends with little time or attention for anything else. To survive the pressure, he reverted to taking the prescription narcotics his neurologist had given him—Tylenol with codeine or Percocet—several nights a week to stave off the pain. A stiff drink at the end of the day had turned into two or three.

Predictably, the drugs and alcohol impaired his ability to think. Focusing on the complexities of his job was a struggle. He slept like a rock but never felt rested. As time went on, he became more irritable. Charlie had always had a friendly and endearing manner with a short fuse. Now the slightest thing set him off.

His father had been a brutal man who had severely battered him as a child. Whatever lingering emotional struggles Charlie carried with him from those violent times, he had been able to step away from them, for the most part, all of these years. His job had given him the comfort of order and structure in his life. In his twenties, he had fallen in love with Suzanne and married her. Although she was devoted to Charlie, she had an emotional detachment he must have welcomed. It made it easier to keep his own emotions safely at bay. With childhood issues of her own, Suzanne had no desire to stir things up.

Two survivors, who had grown up with abuse in place of love, had found each other and made a life together. After years of marriage, there had been no sign that Charlie had inherited a vicious temper from his father. It had always been dormant, but as the months of back pain turned into years, Suzanne was alarmed to see glimpses of it.

Despite his best intentions, Charlie felt increasingly uncooperative and angry. Everyone had always thought of him as a quiet guy who kept to himself, but the mercilessness of the pain was changing him. At work, he would raise his voice and get red in the face over the slightest issue. After watching his behavior closely, Charlie's supervisor accused him of deliberately provoking fights with coworkers. Charlie didn't want that to be true, but he couldn't deny it.

Trying to cope, he started gulping down 50 Excedrin a week. The enormous amount of caffeine in those pills was interfering with his sleep and stressing out his liver and kidneys. The alcohol was only making things worse. He was unquestionably in pain, but where was it coming from? What was he medicating?

MISSING LINKS

We were missing something. Maybe the pain generator was physical, maybe it was psychological. While I was doing multiple workups and imaging studies with Charlie, I began to explore his family history. He gave me more details, describing the regular beatings and violent emotions in the house. All these years of intractable pain couldn't help reminding him of those miserable days as a boy. Here he was again in a dark and hopeless place with no way out.

As he told me about the resentment and anger he still felt toward his father, I explained that freeing himself from these emotional struggles could help alleviate his pain. Sometimes the pain of a traumatic childhood can result in post-traumatic stress disorder, like some soldiers experience after they return from battle.

After feeling hurt and oppressed for as long as he could remember, it had never occurred to Charlie to get help for the chronic emotional pain he felt. When I assured him that he didn't have to feel that way, he agreed to meet with a psychotherapist.

At our regular team meeting, I discussed Charlie's case with his psychotherapist. In all of our patients, we were beginning to notice that previous injury, disease, or emotional trauma was often laying the groundwork for chronic pain. We wondered whether Charlie's back pain was somehow exacerbating the lingering effects of his childhood traumas—or if it was the other way around. Was it possible that his body could remember those assaults at a cellular level and return him to a painful state again, as if it were a set point? Or was his body somehow failing to fight back against this pain because he had been so beaten down as a child?

Increasingly, I observed that the pain patients who had endured traumatic childhoods began to suffer disability in their forties. Their pain became worse and more difficult to control. Depression or anxiety disorders that had been successfully kept at bay increasingly interfered with their lives. It was as if their bodies had endured a heroic struggle to survive, but the battle had taken too high a toll. Some didn't make it to 40 years old. Those who did often found that, as they got older, the traumas they had weathered in the past caught up with them.

I could see the same thing happening with Charlie. No matter what any of his treating physicians or surgeons did, his body seemed to find a way to circumvent our efforts, taking him inexorably back to his original pain.

Eager to get more insight into Charlie's case, I sent him to José Apud, MD, a superb psychopharmacologist. For years Dr. Apud and I had talked frequently about the connection between chronic pain, depression, and trauma. We were seeing an overlap and wanted to know why. Between us, we had received some of the best training in the world, working with some of the most brilliant minds in medicine. Yet the mystery of the connection between chronic pain, depression, and trauma eluded us. The people who suffered from pain and depression seemed to be a different set of people than those who had depression without pain or vice versa. They were all being lumped together.

Like me, Dr. Apud had pursued unusually broad medical training. Maybe we had both known instinctively that we were going to want more answers than a single discipline could provide. There were so many questions, and our knowledge was so limited. It was important to us to be at the cutting edge, where the newest discoveries were being made, so we were constantly cross-fertilizing—going to conferences in psychology, pain, family medicine, nutrition, mind-body medicine, and acupuncture. The only way to solve the mystery was to keep searching.

Hoping to build on my discussions with him, I created a study group to discuss cases, review the latest research, and diligently keep looking for answers. I invited Rosario Nuñez-Brito, MD, to join us. She had done her residency at Georgetown, as I had, and had developed particularly relevant specialties in cognitive-behavioral therapy, psychopharmacology, and post-traumatic stress disorder. Bernardo Hirschman, MD, one of the early members of the study group, brought his expertise in characterological issues. Both of them shared a clinical practice with Dr. Apud. Michael Lumpkin, PhD, the former chairman of the department of physiology at Georgetown Medical School and a specialist in the neurophysiology of stress, rounded out the group. All of us had noticed that our patients who had suffered earlier trauma often developed both chronic pain and depression.

THE LINK BETWEEN PAIN AND DEPRESSION

One of our starting hypotheses was that previous injuries, emotional traumas, and diseases had not just weakened the immune system or "worn down the body"; they had actually primed the body to develop chronic pain and depression many years later. It was not acute pain (like breaking a leg) or situational depression (because a broken leg hurts). The depression was severe, chronic, and inexplicable, just like the pain.

There had to be a reason why chronic pain was so intimately associated with depression. Already, fMRI scans had begun to map areas of the brain that revealed a far more complex interweaving of the emotional and sensory aspects of pain.[12]

What if chronic pain and depression weren't two separate diseases at all? Was it possible they were both part of an unsuspected spectrum disorder?

Studies verified how frequently they came together. Of the estimated 47 million people suffering from chronic pain in America, at least two-thirds of them have a major depressive disorder, too.[13] The likelihood that they would end up permanently disabled—regardless of treatment—was far greater when they had both chronic pain and depression than when they had either one alone.

In ancient Greece, pain was considered to be an emotion, not a sensory experience.[14] Today the International Association for the Study of Pain includes both, defining pain as "an unpleasant sensory and emotional experience."[15] If pain is fundamentally a physical and emotional experience, then it would make sense for an exacerbation of pain to exacerbate emotions, too.

About 52 percent of people with major depressive disorders also suffer from chronic pain. If we flip it the other way, 65 percent of the individuals with chronic pain also suffer from major depressive disorders.[16]

Chronic pain is complex. It's important to assess it from a psychophysiological perspective. Yet most doctors see anxiety, fear, irritability, anger, or depression as unfortunate reactions to pain, rather than elements of the pain itself. Chronic pain is depressing, but that's different from a general state of depression. If a patient is depressed because of the pain (situational depression) and a doctor makes the pain go away, the patient is no longer depressed.

Charlie was depressed even when the pain went away. In fact, when I treated his depression, his back pain got worse. When I alleviated his back pain, his depression got worse. This ping-pong effect was an early clue that made me start wondering whether pain and depression were opposite ends of the same pole. With Charlie I began to suspect for the first time that when it came to pain and depression, we were dealing with a spectrum disorder.

Opening a dialogue about that possibility in the medical community was challenging, since doctors have a tendency to treat physical problems as *real* and emotional repercussions as *unreal*[17] or at best, irrelevant. Yet pain is a predictor of major depression and anxiety. If emotions were irrelevant by-products of pain, why would that be true?

Together, depression and chronic pain dramatically increase the odds of disability. They are also much harder to treat. Each symptom feeds on the other, making it worse. A depressed patient isn't necessarily imagining pain (even if doctors are unable to find an explanation for it), but the bleakness of their perspective creates changes in body chemistry that can make the pain worse—and vice versa.

In the study group, when we looked at the situation more closely, we began to wonder about this combination. When they occurred together, the overlapping pathophysiology looked like a completely different disease process. What if, neurologically, pain and depression were the same thing—at different points on a continuum? Had we been missing the obvious? Was there a pain-depression syndrome? Were pain and emotions different expressions of the same thing?

PHYSICAL EFFECTS OF EMOTION

When Rachel Polson came to see me in her early forties, she'd had chronic pain in her right shoulder for 5 years. X-rays and MRIs had shown no structural damage to her bones or joints, but her shoulder hurt badly enough that she was waking up in the night in pain. When she did sleep through the night, she reported having nightmares and feeling tired when she awoke.

When I examined her, she had myofascial pain syndrome like Charlie did—muscular pain in taut bands with a limited range of motion that did not improve with physical therapy. The patterns of pain radiation were consistent with Dr. Travell's map of the potential trigger points in the body.

Rachel, too, had grown up in a climate of abuse with an alcoholic father and codependent stepmother. Daily traumas—big and small—might well have been routine in a family like that. Then, a few years before I saw her, she was mugged on a dark street, one more physical and emotional assault to add to the rest.

One day, while I was treating her shoulder with osteopathic manual therapy, Rachel began to cry. Images of her attacker flashed vividly through her mind. He had aggressively pushed her down and pinned her to the ground, pressing hardest on her right shoulder, as she tried to fight him off.

Although she'd never really thought about it, her shoulder pain had started sometime after the attack—maybe even months later, as she worked to put it out of her mind. She never saw a therapist, because she believed she had successfully moved past it.

I suggested that her body might still have been holding on to that trauma years later. It certainly couldn't hurt to try counseling to work through it. Whether the pain was lingering for physical or emotional reasons, Rachel wanted to be rid of it, so she did see a therapist. Because her emotional defenses had been strong enough to persuade her that she was over the trauma, it took many sessions over several months to move past them. But when she did, the breakthrough was dramatic. The lightness she felt afterward made her realize she had simply gotten used to carrying a heavy burden. Once she let it go, she was truly free to heal.

She made an appointment to resume the manual therapy on her shoulder. Without the emotional lock on the pain of the past, her body was available for recovery. This time, when we addressed the pain generators in her muscles, they responded and the pain finally went away. In retrospect, the situation was easy to assess.

As we've said, the body has such a limited range of expression when it comes to pain. It doesn't distinguish well between physical and emotional pain. With its capacity to hold on to old traumas, it barely distinguishes between the past and the present.

We didn't yet know why, but it was becoming obvious that, when remnants of old wounds were left unresolved, they were building up inside the body. But the traumas were not just cumulative—one added to the other. When they cropped up again, they did it in synergy, an effect much greater than the sum of the parts. The pain manifesting in Rachel's shoulder was far too deep to be treated with manual therapy alone. The muscles and the fascia were almost like the overflow valve for the pressure that was building elsewhere.

Out of our ignorance in the medical profession, we have done a disservice to patients like Rachel by stigmatizing this kind of pain as "psychosomatic." Her chronic shoulder pain was not imaginary. The treatment that resolved it was not purely psychological, because the pain was not entirely physiological, either. A psychophysiological process was at work.

We have wrongly assumed that emotions cannot induce physiological changes. If doctors condescend to patients when the origins of their pain are based on emotional rather than physical traumas, it is because we have not understood the nature of pain.

PAIN BEFORE INJURY

In his work in rehabilitation at the New York University School of Medicine, John Sarno, MD, found that pain did not always have a physical cause. In fact, it was far more likely to be caused by specific emotions.

It is our medical bias to look for mechanical or structural causes. If a patient presents with back pain, the only valid explanation, for most doctors, is physical: a football injury, a car accident, a saggy bed. When an emotional trauma—the loss of a loved one, a frustrating marriage, or a burden of guilt—results in pain, doctors tend to treat it like a mental problem. If no mechanical or structural issue can be found, the patient's pain must be "in his head." A doctor may refer the patient to a psychologist but not without a hint of contempt, as if psychophysiological pain were a sign of poor character at best, mental illness at worst.

The idea that pain is primarily caused by injury or physical damage has been deeply ingrained in all of us. Dr. Sarno wrote: "I have never seen a patient with pain in the neck, shoulders, back or buttocks who didn't believe that the pain was due to an injury . . . brought on by some physical activity. 'I hurt myself while running (playing basketball, tennis, bowling).' 'Ten years ago I was involved in a hit-from-behind auto accident and I have had recurrent back pain ever since.' "[18]

If the pain starts in relation to a physical activity or trauma, it's logical to attribute the pain to that incident. It may be just as logical to attribute pain to an emotional stressor or trauma, but emotions are much harder to test in a laboratory.[19]

In fact, the body may not discriminate between emotional and physical trauma in any significant way. When we understand the relationship between emotions and pain more fully, we may even find, as Dr. Sarno believes, that many of the conditions we have assumed to have structural causes—such as herniated discs, pinched nerves, arthritis, bone spurs, and plantar fasciitis—have very specific emotional precursors. Until we remove the stigma from emotional origins of pain, we stand little chance at being able to objectively explore the connection.

I was beginning to notice that when chronic pain was the issue, the cause was rarely a single thing. It was an accumulation of things. Unfortunately, the underlying mechanism that united all of these events in the body still eluded us.

A series of assaults may very well not result in chronic pain. Sometimes it didn't; sometimes it did. Until we knew what was making the difference, we didn't really know what was going on. We could only say that somehow an accumulation of physical or emotional assaults was overwhelming the body—in some cases—leaving it vulnerable, hypersensitive to pain. It wasn't an answer, but it gave us something to explore.

Chronic pain often appeared to start with a thing, an incident that triggered peripheral pain generators, but on close examination, it would always turn out to be more complicated than that. People talk about picking up a pair of socks and having their back go out. As a doctor, my job is to ask: How did we get here? What were all the things that led up to this? Picking up socks should not put you on the floor in pain. Assuming your back cannot go out "suddenly" because you bent over, what really happened?

Maybe everyday stress caused you to hold tension in your muscles. Instead of massaging it away or doing exercises to release the stress, you ignored it and kept going. Maybe your bed sagged and your chair was off ergonomically, so your muscles were in a subtle but constant strain all night and all day. In the afternoon, your back was a little sore after you worked out at the gym or raced around the park with your kids.

Then one day, emotional stress upped the ante. At work, your boss or client was demanding. Construction on the road made your commute a nightmare. By the time you got home, you were unusually tense. Your shoulders were tight. The muscles in your back, your neck, and all the way down your arms were trying to compensate, doing things they weren't designed to do. But you didn't notice, because when you finally got home, something happened to push your body over the edge.

It might have been a little annoyance. It might have been more serious. Almost certainly, it had nothing to do with socks. But when you reached to pick them up off the floor, your back couldn't take it anymore. All those little strains caught up with you, and you were in pain.

Pain is always the result of trauma, either physical or psychological—or very commonly, both. When the pain becomes chronic, we must look for all the cumulative events that led up to this. What isn't allowing the body to heal?

A PING-PONG EFFECT

When I saw Charlie again in 1995, therapy had been very helpful for his marriage, and he was no longer drinking. The fundamental issues of his childhood abuse, however, had still not been addressed. His back pain continued to plague him. Charlie even commented that it seemed as if he had a choice between pain or depression because when one got better the other always seemed to get worse. It was a very bad sign.

It was a pattern I'd seen before, a kind of ping-pong effect. As the psychological issues getter better, the pain gets worse, and vice versa. It's a perpetually unstable state. It worried me to see that pattern in Charlie because I knew it was impossible to sustain. Every time the emotional pain pings back to the physical pain and back again, it wears down the body's resilience.

Soon my treatments were having a diminishing effect. What had worked for him in the past wasn't able to hold back the pain anymore. He went back to therapy again, but felt dissatisfied and changed psychotherapists several times. He felt exhausted yet couldn't sleep. Nothing seemed to be helping.

Eight long years passed, as Charlie went from doctor to doctor, looking for answers. By 2003, things had gotten so much worse that he couldn't work and was at the brink of taking a permanent disability leave from Halliburton. He came to me in desperation.

Charlie said he'd had surgery for his back pain, but it hadn't helped. I couldn't imagine what the surgeon had done, since he had no nerve damage, no disc damage, no instability of the spine. His scans had all been normal. Most practitioners would agree that pain was not an indication for surgery. In fact, it was very likely a contraindication.

Charlie's pain had temporarily subsided after surgery, which is not uncommon as a placebo response, but then it intensified until it was far worse than before. Gradually, his condition had degenerated to a level he would never have expected. His back pain had steadily increased until it dominated his thoughts. All day long at work, he based his decisions—about where to sit, when to take a break, how often to get up and walk around—on the amount of pain he was in. His ability to concentrate had seriously declined.

After so many years, I reluctantly prescribed narcotic pain medication. At the time, extended-release opioids were already the standard of care for cancer-related pain and were being cautiously recommended for benign (noncancerous) chronic pain.[20] It was thought that opioids could be an effective treatment for all kinds of pain, regardless of their pathophysiological mechanism.[21] The sad fact was that, for some people, nothing else worked. If they were to have any hope of controlling their pain and returning to some semblance of a productive life, narcotics were their only option.

With the use of narcotics, there was, of course, a concern about addiction. To help alleviate this concern, the medical community made a nuanced distinction between *addiction* and *dependency.*

Virtually everyone we put on narcotics became dependent on them to reduce their pain to tolerable levels. So the term *dependency* became a way to acknowledge that everyone would have withdrawal symptoms when they stopped taking the drug. *Addiction,* by contrast, was defined, not as physical withdrawal, but as a pattern of behavior associated with drug seeking and a patient's need for increasing amounts of the drug to go beyond pain control and get high. It was a very fine line.

We could do nothing about dependency, but we did attempt to reduce the chances of addiction. After I discussed the use and side effects of the medication with Charlie, I had him sign a narcotic contract. It stated that he understood the benefits and risks of the medication, that he would not get the medication from anyone else, that he would take it only as prescribed, and that he would agree to random drug testing, so we would know he was taking the medication accordingly.

We noticed that after several months on narcotics, Charlie's depression was worsening, but without it, his pain was unbearable. So we looked for another solution.

The study group recommended consultations with neurologists and anesthesiologists. One of them tried the dorsal column stimulator (DCS), invented by my mentor, Dr. Norm Shealy. It stimulated the spinal cord with electrodes to block the pain signal. With Charlie, it alleviated the pain enough that we could reduce the dose of his narcotics, which helped alleviate his depression.

But the years of enduring such a low quality of life had taken their toll. Despite years of our best efforts, Charlie took an early retirement from Halliburton at 50 years old and moved closer to Suzanne's family in Santa Fe, where she took care of him.

It was a devastating result, but the truth was, we couldn't help him, because we simply didn't know enough yet. After watching what happened to Charlie, I was more determined than ever to understand this perplexing phenomenon. What was the connection between chronic pain and emotional pain?

We still didn't know exactly what chronic pain was. If we were completely honest with ourselves, we didn't really know what depression was either. Both of these conditions obviously had severe consequences. Both presented together a majority of the time. And yet we still had no biologic markers to diagnose individuals who suffered from them. No blood test or brain scan would show anything we could identify. Or so it seemed.

Part II
Solving the Mystery

Chapter 4

EUREKA!

DISCOVERING THE SINGLE POINT OF ORIGIN

Discoveries are made by giving attention
to the slightest clue.

William I. B. Beveridge

Tucking a wisp of blond hair behind her ear, Nicole de Laive gazed out the tinted plate-glass windows of a high-rise. To her right, a tower in the unlikely but instantly identifiable shape of a blue gherkin gleamed in the sun. She recognized the angular brown box of St. Helen's next door. And that was Tower 42 in the distance. Apparently, she was in the City—London's financial district—probably the Willis Building, which meant she could stop by that great little bar on Broad Street while she was here, if she had the time.

The sun was just beginning to set, but that didn't mean anything. If this was November—and she suspected it was—twilight would kick off around 3:30 p.m. In these northern latitudes, the light disappeared so early, you could never tell what time it was. She glanced at her watch.

"Nicole?"

Startled by the voice, she turned. Fifteen executives in finely tailored suits sat waiting at a conference table. *What on earth am I doing here?* Smiling defensively, Nicole took a firm step forward on her Ferragamo pumps. A glance at the whiteboard told her what she'd been up to. All the notes and arrows were in her handwriting.

"Just checking to see how much time we have," she explained.

Nicole was a high-powered consultant, able to walk into any office, find the problem, fix it, and walk out again for a handsome remuneration. This was the kind of thing she did from LA to Brussels, and she worked with the best.

So it was odd that she couldn't seem to remember who these people were or what she might have been saying that, judging by the state of the conference table, had given them time to go through numerous cups of coffee and almost 20 pages of her prospectus. Her mind sprinted to catch up. If this was the Willis Building, these were probably Boyd & Hastings execs. She'd evaluated their reports last week and set up a meeting to discuss her findings. *Was this that meeting?*

She would have to assume it was. Indisputably a type-A personality, Nicole had always been in the fast lane, moving ahead, taking control, striving harder. She was certainly not going to let a little thing like a memory lapse embarrass her in front of important clients.

Moving confidently to the head of the table, she looked the executives in the eye and said, "So. Where were we?"

For the first time in her career, Nicole's confidence was an absolute bluff.

SLIPPING AWAY

After finishing the job at Boyd & Hastings, Nicole tried to reduce the number of hours she was working. She told herself that she'd been working too hard and just needed a good rest. Despite her considerable ability to compartmentalize her concerns, nagging fears kept creeping up from the back of her mind. It was 2009. Like it or not, she was 50. *What if this was menopause? Or early-onset Alzheimer's?*

Whatever it was, it got worse before it got better.

One night someone tried to break into her mother-in-law's house. Although no one managed to get in, Nicole and her husband, Rick, were greatly disturbed. Realizing how vulnerable Rick's mother was as a 95-year-old woman who lived alone, they worked to double-secure all the entries and scheduled a locksmith to come and change all the locks.

The very next day, when Rick asked Nicole to follow up with the locksmith, she didn't know what he was talking about. Nicole had no memory at all of the attempted break-in the night before.

One bright Sunday afternoon at home, Nicole pulled the duvet and sheets off the bed. Lugging armloads of bedding to the washer, she joked with Rick and his friends as they settled onto the sofas to watch the playoffs. A few hours later, she took the dry sheets back and made up the bed.

When the game ended, they all had tapas and beer together, then Rick's friends went home in the early evening. It had been a long, enjoyable day. As their guests were leaving, Nicole thought how great it would be to sleep on crisp white sheets. So she stripped off the bedding and lugged it to the washer.

Rick stopped her in the middle of the room. "What are you doing?"

"It's okay. They have time to dry before we go to bed and then we can sleep on nice fresh sheets!"

"You did those this morning."

Nicole frowned. "Are you sure?"

"You walked right by us. Are you okay?"

As her brain lapses became more common, Rick and Nicole tried to diffuse the awkwardness by making light of it. "Looks like you screwed the pooch again!" Rick would say affectionately, giving her a hug, and Nicole would laugh. But both of them were worried.

Simple things were becoming difficult. Nicole would drive across town on an errand and forget what it was before she got there. She would take a shower and leave the water running.

At first, the damages were minimal, but that didn't last. She was frying fish in a hot skillet one night when her mind wandered and she walked out of the room. Ten minutes later, the smoke alarm went off. The high-pitched squeal sent her running back into the kitchen. Until she saw the sizzling skillet, she had no idea why the smoke alarm had gone off. She didn't even remember starting dinner.

Rick tried to assure her that it could happen to anyone, but Nicole knew better. She could feel herself slipping away.

A few weeks later, she could barely walk. She woke up one morning and staggered to the bathroom as if she were drunk. She had to brace herself against the doorframe to keep from tumbling onto the tile floor. It should have been alarming, but she couldn't get her mind to focus. She felt confused, disoriented. She made it to the toilet but couldn't stand back up. Her body wouldn't function. She felt as if she were in the middle of a seizure and all of her muscles had locked. Rick had to help her back to bed.

The next day, they made an emergency appointment at the Kaplan Center and got in to see Lisa Lilienfield, the doctor on our team who specializes in women's medicine. Dr. Lisa examined her and ran some tests. While they were waiting for the results, she sent Nicole to a neurologist.

When the MRI scan revealed damage to her brain, the neurologist diagnosed her with multiple sclerosis.

No one knows what causes it, but multiple sclerosis (MS) begins with sustained inflammation of the brain and spinal cord that eventually damages the myelin sheath (the outgrowth of glial cells that serves as protective insulation around the nerves). Other conditions can produce similar symptoms, but when they're accompanied by inflammatory damage like this, it usually means MS. Neuropsychological testing also showed cognitive and memory issues so severe that she was designated totally disabled.

The prognosis was dismal. Nicole had already experienced many of the symptoms: loss of memory, difficulty walking or moving her arms and legs, poor coordination, and muscular weakness. But MS is neurodegenerative. If she had it, the medical literature said she could expect an irreversible decline in her ability to function or even control her own movements. At that point, she could get assistance—from physical therapists, speech therapists, and social workers or gadgets, walkers, and wheelchairs—but her condition would get steadily worse. And there is no known cure.[1]

A LESSER EVIL

Nicole was still trying to grasp the fact that life as she'd known it was never going to be the same, when Dr. Lisa called.

"When can I see you?" Dr. Lisa said. "The blood tests just came back. You've got Lyme disease, from a deer tick, apparently."

"A deer tick? I work 80 hours a week in an office. I drive from my garage to my clients' garages and back! How could a tick have bitten me?"

"I don't know," Dr. Lisa laughed. "But the test results are clear. We still can't rule out multiple sclerosis at this time, but we know that Lyme disease mimics MS. If we have a specialist treat you for Lyme and you get better, we may be able to dismiss the diagnosis of MS altogether."

Given the option, Nicole would have vastly preferred Lyme disease over MS, but she was still a long way from getting well. On top of the memory loss, she still had a bad shake that made her feel like an elderly woman. If she looked to the right, she couldn't see out of either eye. Her eyes were fine, but apparently there was damage to her brain precisely where the optical nerves crossed. The entire right side of her body felt numb.

Dr. Lisa referred her to an infectious disease specialist, who put her on an intravenous antibiotic, Rocephin, for 28 days. For 26 of those days, Nicole didn't walk so much as stagger. Her balance was impaired and her muscles were not always willing to respond to her commands.

With 2 days of antibiotics left, she got up from the sofa and walked to the kitchen without jerking and stumbling across the room. When Rick applauded, as if she were a toddler taking her first steps, she felt a flush of embarrassment. And then tears came to her eyes. It was one of the earliest signs that she was getting better.

The antibiotics were finally beginning to work. She felt the first glimmer of hope. If she could keep taking them a little longer, maybe they would completely resolve the problem! They certainly might have helped, but her doctor stopped the antibiotics, saying that the CDC recommended against the use of intravenous antibiotics after 28 days. He told her nothing more could be done for her.

After the disappointment sunk in, Nicole tried again. She found what the Lyme community calls an LLMD, a Lyme-literate doctor, who continued to treat her, but she did not seem to get better. She still felt very confused. Her memory was appalling. She still had tremors throughout the day, and the right side of her body was numb.

SHATTERED HOPE

And then one day, she met her brother, Paul, for lunch. They had been talking and laughing throughout the meal. Everything seemed fine. Nicole waved good-bye as Paul drove away, and then she couldn't find her car. A feeling of panic rose up in the pit of her stomach as she looked around the parking lot. Had her car been stolen? She started to call the police, but, remembering the incident with the laundry, she called her brother instead.

"Stay where you are," Paul said. "I'm on my way back."

Nicole waited. About 10 minutes later, when Paul pulled up next to her and parked his car, he had a funny look on his face. "What is it?" she said.

"Isn't that your car?" Paul pointed to her black BMW convertible, not 10 feet away from where she was standing.

A few weeks later, when Nicole went to the grocery store, the same thing happened again. She thought her car was not where she'd parked it. This time, when she started to panic, she took a deep breath and tried to stay calm. With all of her groceries, she walked back into the grocery store and turned around. "Let's try this again," she told herself.

This time, when she walked back out into the parking lot, she found her car but didn't like what she saw. Her car had rolled out of its parking space and into another car. Apparently, she'd forgotten to set the brake. Nicole had been driving manual transmissions for 35 years and had never forgotten to set the brake before.

Nicole went back to Dr. Lisa the next day and said, "I don't stagger anymore, and that's great. But I can't do anything else! When my memory is so bad I can't remember how to park my car, how can I work? Will I even remember how to get to a client's office?"

Dr. Lisa sent Nicole back to the neurologist, who requested that the extensive neuropsychological testing be redone to see if there was any improvement. The results showed no improvement, but she hadn't gotten worse.

As the months wore on, the strain was almost too much for Nicole. She was not able to do some of the easiest, most basic things. On top of everything else, she felt she was letting Rick down. They had planned for him to retire the year she got sick, but, with Nicole unable to work, Rick had to keep working. And they didn't know how long it would have to go on.

The situation was so discouraging that Nicole was crying all the time. Her confident business consultant persona was gone. She spent most of her days feeling worthless and defeated.

Seeing how miserable she was, everyone encouraged her to take antidepressants. She tried them for a month, but they didn't help. Dr. Lisa asked her to see the therapist at the Kaplan Center for at least 6 weeks.

After meeting with Nicole a few times, the therapist canceled the rest of the sessions. "You're not depressed," she said. "You're upset and pissed off about the horrible situation you're in. Who wouldn't be?"

MEETING NICOLE

At that point, Nicole was referred to me. Because of our biweekly meetings to discuss patients at the clinic, I was already aware of her case.

She had been diagnosed with and treated for Lyme with only a partial response to therapy. What were we missing? After reviewing the reports of the other physicians and taking Nicole's history myself, I ran blood tests for heavy metals.

The first test came back negative. I explained to Nicole that if she did have heavy metal toxicity and the test was negative, the metals were not actively circulating in her blood. Another test would tell us if they were being harbored in her bones and tissue.

The results of the second test showed that Nicole had a significant amount of lead in her tissues. Lead, mercury, arsenic, and other heavy metals are ubiquitous in our environment, and there are many potential sources of poisoning. Heavy metals poison many enzyme systems in the body and can cause a number of illnesses, but they especially damage our nerves and brain.

Nicole had suffered from lead poisoning as a child after eating paint chips, but she was unsure whether she had ever been treated. That episode and decades of exposure to the fumes from leaded gasoline left me suspicious that heavy metals, festering in her tissues, were interfering with her recovery.

Treating the whole patient often requires careful decisions about which issues to address first. Despite the standard recommendations of the CDC in general, recent studies have shown that more than 20 percent of people with Lyme develop what the CDC calls post-treatment Lyme disease syndrome (PTLDS).[2] In those people, Lyme persists after treatment, evading the standard course of antibiotics.[3] Because of this, the duration and type of antibiotic treatment must be tailored to each patient. Many physicians believe that treatment for Lyme must continue until the patient has been symptom free for at least a month.

One of the concerns is that when patients develop PTLDS, it is because some unseen factor is suppressing their immune system, inhibiting their recovery. In Nicole's case, I wondered if the elevated lead levels in her body were creating that effect. Lead poisoning could have been responsible for some of her symptoms, and it might also have been keeping her from recovering from Lyme.

The treatment for Nicole's lead poisoning could be handled quickly with chelation therapy, which might relieve her symptoms, as well as improve her immune function, but we could not do it while she was taking antibiotics. So I took her off the antibiotics, treated her for lead poisoning with oral chelation therapy, then put her back on antibiotics for Lyme.

As the months went by, Nicole's memory gradually began to come back. The shaking became more moderate. The area of numbness on her right side began to diminish as well, proving it had never been multiple sclerosis.

"If this had gone much further," Nicole said, "I think I would've been in a wheelchair for life."

After she finished the second course of antibiotics, I put her on Atacand, a blood pressure medication, and low-dose naltrexone to quell the inflammation. My research indicated that the inflammation in the brain caused by Lyme and Lyme-related diseases could not be reduced by antibiotics and antiparasitic medications alone.

I prescribed low-dose Naltrexone, a very versatile medication. It is used in emergency rooms to save the lives of patients who have overdosed on drugs. By counteracting the addictive high of morphine, heroin, and alcohol, it has also given substance abusers relief from their addictions. My research has shown that Naltrexone acts to reduce inflammation in the brain. That makes it useful in treating conditions such as fibromyalgia and Lyme-related diseases, where antibiotics alone do not result in total recovery.

THE PRACTICE OF PARTIAL RECOVERY

If it was already obvious in medical school that people were suffering from increasingly complicated conditions, it was even worse now. The patients we saw at the clinic had often seen 8 to 15 other physicians before coming to the center. It was not uncommon for them to have been evaluated and treated at some of our best medical centers such as Mayo Clinic and Johns Hopkins. We were still able to help most of the people who came to see us, but achieving total recovery was proving more elusive.

The underlying mechanism was still a mystery. And I knew that until we found the cause, we would never find a cure.

With our patients exhibiting such a wide array of symptoms, it was nearly impossible to see the connection. How were physical injuries, viral infections, nutritional deficits, hormonal imbalances, and emotional disorders related? What was the common denominator?

Again and again, my mind kept returning to the common occurrence of pain and depression in the same people. Some of the people who experienced chronic pain may already have been prone to mood disorders, of course. For others, the persistent physical misery of chronic pain may have given way to a feeling of despair. But even taking those two possibilities into account, the number of people who had both pain and depression was inexplicably high.

In the general population, approximately 16 percent will experience a major bout of depression in their lives, while 15 percent will experience chronic pain in any given year. Of those people, 65 percent will experience both at the same time.[4]

There was also a growing recognition that people who had both conditions together had a dramatically lower chance of recovery with our current treatments. The odds of recovering from a major bout of depression were 47 percent. If a patient had both pain and depression, the likelihood of recovery dropped precipitously to 9 percent.[5]

It was obvious *what* was happening, but *why* was it happening?

DIGGING DEEPER

Dr. José Apud and I often had long conversations, wondering what it was that brought our specialties—pain management and psychiatry—together so frequently. As new research would come out, we would pour over it in the study group, looking for clues that could explain the connection between these two conditions.

Judging by the deterioration I was seeing in the patients who arrived at my clinic, I was starting to suspect that both pain and depression were neurodegenerative. But I was spending hours reading medical journals, and none of the literature was talking about it.

It was slowly dawning on me that if I was determined to isolate the underlying mechanisms of these conditions, I was going to have to go deeper into neurophysiology than I'd expected. In medical school, I'd originally planned to become a neurologist. Now it looked like I was going to end up going down that road after all. Compiling all the latest studies on neuroinflammation in depression, I dug in, assuming I was going to have to put myself through a mini-master's program in neurophysiology before I found anything that could help the patients with complicated conditions.

Months went by. Each time I found something of interest, I would take it to the group or discuss it with Dr. Apud, but I didn't find anything too enlightening at first.

Late one night, I came across a paper by neurologist Michael J. Robinson and his colleagues at Eli Lilly, one of the largest pharmaceutical companies in the world. Examining pain and depression from a neurological point of view, he found they had more in common than the medical community had assumed. In fact, they shared much of the same neurophysiology. More exciting, however, were his arguments that these were both neuroinflammatory diseases.[6]

This was a breakthrough insight. I rushed the data to the study group, and we set to work, trying to grasp the implications. Two questions were foremost in my mind:

- If pain and depression shared a similar neurological base, were they two separate diseases or different manifestations of the same disease?
- And when they occurred together, what made them ignite a synergy, creating a condition that was more than the sum of its parts?

The idea that pain and depression were inflammatory diseases was a radically new concept. It would require a completely different approach than either physicians or psychiatrists had been using to evaluate and treat patients.

In 2009, we understood very little about the nature of inflammation in the central nervous system. The brain is considered "an immunologically privileged" organ. Our brains have their own unique immune systems. While the brain's immune system can and does interact with the peripheral immune system, that interaction is limited and closely regulated.

The brain and spinal cord, which make up the central nervous system (CNS), are connected to every organ and limb by the peripheral nervous system. Because of its vital importance, the CNS is completely encased in bone. From the top of our skulls to the base our spines, it is shielded from external assaults. Deep inside, our brains are protected from contamination by the blood-brain barrier. As R. Douglas Fields explains in

The Other Brain, "The cells forming the walls of blood vessels in the central nervous system are sealed together so tightly that cells and molecules in the bloodstream, which freely pass into tissue elsewhere in the body, are unable to cross into brain tissue."[7] It was widely assumed that because of this barrier, brain inflammation was rare, the result of extreme illnesses or violent injuries.

Curiously enough, the response of patients with hepatitis was raising questions about these assumptions. When they were treated with interferon, these patients consistently became clinically depressed.[8] Since interferon is one of the molecules that causes inflammation in the body, researchers came to suspect that there was an undiscovered link between inflammation and depression.

In the last few years, as they began to investigate, they discovered that anxiety disorders and PTSD also accompanied elevated inflammatory molecules in the central nervous system. This led to the astonishing conclusion that depression, anxiety, and PTSD were all neuroinflammatory diseases in the brain.[9]

It is important to clarify what we mean when we talk about inflammation. There are many different types of inflammatory pathways in the body. When we call all of them "inflammation," it's like talking generally about "illness." Physiologically, each type of inflammation is very different, engaging different types of cells and different parts of the immune system.

At the simplest level, inflammation associated with allergies is mediated by one pathway (IgE), food intolerances by another (IgG), and celiac disease by others (IgA and IgG anti-tTG). Bacterial infections cause inflammation by a completely different route (the activation of white cells), while biotoxic inflammation involves cytokines and interferon.

We may use an antibiotic to treat the inflammation from a bacterial infection, but the same antibiotic would be completely ineffective in treating an allergic response, just as the antihistamines or steroids we might use to treat an allergy would do little to combat bacteria.

What we're just beginning to understand is that inflammation quickly gets complicated. Depending on how many cumulative traumas the body has endured, inflammation can spread like a brush fire. When it flares up in one pathway, it can ignite a secondary inflammatory response in peripheral pathways.

Inflammation has been a hot topic in medicine for the last 10 years. Within the integrative medical community, many chronic diseases are being seen as a consequence of chronic inflammation throughout the body. New studies are confirming neurodegeneration that is the result of sustained low-grade inflammatory states. There is speculation that central nervous system inflammation may be a precursor to all kinds of conditions, from autism to fibromyalgia to Alzheimer's.[10] It is even thought that inflammation in the spinal cord may be a mechanism for chronic pain.[11]

In 2009, Dr. Robinson and his team were among the early researchers to connect both pain and depression to inflammation in the brain. If they were right that pain and depression were neuroinflammatory diseases with a common origin, the real question was: What was causing and sustaining that inflammation?

FINDING THE CONNECTION

While I was mulling it over, I attended a seminar at the American Academy of Pain Management about inflammatory factors in the brain—interleukins, a group of signaling molecules that participate in the body's immune responses, and the tiny cells that would change my whole way of thinking: microglia.

The more I read about microglia, the more I was convinced that they played an important role in the development of pain and depression.

Microglia act as the resident immune system of the central nervous system. If anything manages to slip past the blood-brain barrier, the microglia intervene. "Squeezing between tangles of dendrites and axons as they rush to kill the invader, microglia attack and devour any harmful organism."[12]

In order to protect the brain, the microglia secrete inflammatory chemicals to create swelling that acts as a buffer, as they work to destroy the invaders. While this inflammatory counterattack is going on at the molecular level, the person enduring it begins to feel sick with fatigue, headaches, fevers, and achiness all over.

As I began to investigate microglia, I found dozens of articles in medical journals, each one linking microglial inflammation to a different stressor: physical injury, psychological trauma, loss of oxygen to the brain, bacterial infections, viral infections, environmental toxins—the list was long. Whenever the central nervous system was stressed, the microglia upregulated, responding the only way they knew how: by creating inflammation.

And suddenly I saw it.

When microglia are upregulated, they create widespread inflammation in the central nervous system. If they are turned on too often, they become hyperreactive, keeping the brain in a chronic state of inflammation.

In some people, the microglia remain activated for longer periods of time. We see evidence of this in teenagers who binge drink. Heavy alcohol consumption triggers the microglia. Researchers in one study confirmed that teenagers' nervous systems were measurably inflamed, then checked their levels of inflammation at intervals to see when it subsided. (Inflammatory chemicals, Interleukin-6, TNF alpha, and Interleukin-1 beta are clear biomarkers for upregulation of microglia because they are produced by microglia in the brain.) After the teenagers stopped drinking, their microglia remained upregulated for a decade.[13]

What this study demonstrates is two very important concepts. The first is that the traumas we suffer have a cumulative effect. Every injury, every infection, every toxin, every physical trauma, every emotional blow generates the same reaction. Inside the brain, it triggers the microglia again and again and again.

The second realization is even more startling. There comes a point when the microglia have been activated in such a way that they remain upregulated, continuing to spew out inflammatory chemicals even though the trauma that originally caused them to become active is no longer present. That response can show up in any number of ways: chronic pain, depression, anxiety disorders, fibromyalgia, chronic headaches, and

PTSD, to name a few. All of these and many other medical conditions are the manifestation of chronic microglia activation.

No matter how it shows up, any condition that is caused by the activation of microglia is just a variation on the theme. Genetic proclivities or the particular combination of cumulative assaults result in different manifestations, but at the physiological level, one single underlying process is taking place.

Now I had a target, a way of understanding inflammation in the central nervous system. My first goal was to identify everything that makes the microglia start setting fires in the brain. Treating those things would surely improve my patients' conditions.

The second goal would be to understand how to turn off the microglia and return them to their non-inflammatory resting state once their job of protecting the brain from the original trauma was completed.

But the implications were even greater than that. Medicine was getting it all wrong. Chronic pain in all its forms—depression, PTSD, and a number of other neuropsychiatric conditions—were not distinct diseases but symptoms of an underlying neuroinflammatory disease. The cause of that inflammation was chronically upregulated microglia.

This was the underlying mechanism I'd been searching for, the common denominator behind all of these symptoms.

Now it made sense that Billy could develop an extreme disease like reflex sympathetic dystrophy after a leak in the basement and a sports injury. For Emily, it had started with severe physical injuries in a car accident, compounded by repeated surgeries, pain medications, and severe psychological stress. With Charlie, a repetitive series of events—physical and psychological abuse as a child, sports traumas, surgeries, myofascial damage, alcohol abuse, and even some of the medications meant to address his pain—had tipped the scales.

All of these events had seemed unrelated, but all of them upregulate microglia in exactly the same way. With the body's limited range of expression, the reaction isn't nuanced. Whatever the assault, it's on/off like a toggle switch.

With repeated assaults, the microglia in the brain become hyperreactive. If the inflammation never subsides, even a minor injury can make pain chronic long after the original injury has healed. The injury is only the tipping point.

In excitement over this *Eureka!* moment, my mind was leaping ahead to connect the dots. The implications were profound. It proved, in an entirely new way, that disease is the outcome of our life experiences.

HUMBLING INSIGHTS

In medical science, it is not unusual to spend a lot of time getting it wrong before we get it right. "The genius of the scientific method, however, is that it accepts no permanent solution. Skepticism is its solvent, for every theory is imperfect. Scientific facts are meaningful precisely because they are ephemeral, because a new observation, a more honest observation, can always alter them."[14]

In the meantime, we are always certain about what we know until we are certain we know something else.

Once we make a discovery, it's not uncommon for years to go by before anyone brings it to the public. As William Beveridge reminds us in his classic book *The Art of Scientific Investigation*, "Edward Jenner was not the first to inoculate people with cowpox to protect them against smallpox, William Harvey was not the first to postulate circulation of the blood, Darwin was by no means the first to suggest evolution, Columbus was not the first European to go to America, Pasteur was not the first to propound the germ theory of disease, Lister was not the first to use carbolic acid as a wound antiseptic."[15] These were the people who made the idea available to what William Beveridge called the "reluctant world."[16] There is a certain natural resistance to new ideas, even when they represent exciting changes that will shape the future for the better.

Few ideas are original. Usually they have a history. More often than not, someone else—often several people—previously suggested something very much like it. That's why Steve Jobs said that people who come up with the ideas feel reluctant to say they invented something new.

With every new insight, we are inevitably amazed and humbled by how often we get even the basic things wrong. All we can do is keep searching for answers, knowing each one will open the door to new insights.

In 2013, President Barack Obama announced the Brain Research through Advancing Innovative Neurotechnologies (BRAIN) Initiative, designed to map the human brain for the first time, saying, "The BRAIN Initiative will accelerate the development and application of new technologies that will enable researchers to produce dynamic pictures of the brain that show how individual brain cells and complex neural circuits interact at the speed of thought."[17] In 2006, the Human Brain Project was launched in Europe in order to employ supercomputing technology to build brain models of any species at any stage in its development. Already the project has successfully built a detailed model of one of the brain's building blocks: the neocortical column.[18] With the United States and the European Union devoting billions of dollars to mapping the brain, we may soon understand previously incomprehensible aspects of brain function.

When scientists got their earliest look at the cells in the brain with the development of new microscopes more than 100 years ago, what they discovered astonished them. As R. Douglas Fields reported in *Scientific American*, "Brain cells were unlike those anywhere else in the body. Their observations revolutionized our understanding of the brain and charted the course of neuroscience for the next century."[19]

Since then, scientists have employed electrodes and imaging technologies to study how small networks of neurons respond to stimuli, but our brains have 100 billion neurons, engaged in complex interactions. As of yet, no technology exists with the speed or resolution to track these movements.[20]

Initially, microglia were dismissed as "housekeeping cells," cleaning up the debris in the brain. Until 1991, one of the leading medical school textbooks stated unequivocally that "microglia have become the most controversial element of the central nervous system; indeed, their very existence is in doubt."[21]

These recent discoveries about microglia are so new they haven't had time to show up in textbooks yet. We now know that glial cells not only sense electrical activity flowing through neural circuits, but they can also control it. Glia are involved in every part of health or disease in the central nervous system.[22] Studies show that a variety of pathologies can activate microglia, including traumatic brain injury, hypoxia, ischemia, physical or emotional trauma, emotional stress, bacterial and viral infections, absorption of environmental toxins such as lead or diesel-exhaust particles, and neurodegenerative diseases such as Alzheimer's, Parkinson's, multiple sclerosis, and AIDS-related dementia.

Our cerebral cortex—where all of our "big thinking" occurs—makes up 80 percent of the brain's mass. Of that mass, only 17 percent of the cells are neurons, and all the rest (83 percent) are glial cells. It stands to reason that the glia may play a more important role than we previously imagined.[23]

There is a growing body of evidence that microglia "remember" prior assaults. Once they are activated, they set off inflammation throughout the nervous system. When the body returns to normal, they return to a resting state until the next time the body is assaulted. With repeated assaults over time, the microglia appear to ramp up, activating more quickly with each assault and becoming more reluctant to return to a resting state.

We are only beginning to understand this function of the brain. At this early stage, it seems that long-term activation of microglia may play a key role in creating and sustaining the kind of complicated chronic pain and depression conditions that appear to be on the rise.

With these insights, three things already seem certain:

- Chronic pain and depression are inflammatory and neurodegenerative conditions.
- Tiny cells in the brain, called microglia, are the source of that inflammation.
- Physical and emotional traumas in our lives are not unrelated. Together, they have a cumulative effect on our bodies' inflammation.

THE COST OF UNRESOLVED TRAUMA

While I was mulling over these realizations, a new patient came to my office. Now 32 years old, Kelly had been diagnosed with fibromyalgia at the age of 20. Since that time, she had struggled with brain fog, sleep disturbances, headaches, PMS, and sensitivity to changes in temperature, loud noises, and bright lights. Her body was hyperreactive to pain.

According to the National Institutes of Health, fibromyalgia is common, but its causes are still unknown. It can arise after a physical or emotional trauma, repetitive injuries, or illness, but sometimes it appears to occur spontaneously. It is thought to reflect a problem in the way the central nervous system processes pain.[24]

As always, I asked Kelly to describe her entire medical history. She began by telling me she had suffered a minor concussion from a car accident when she was 18. Two years later, her health had deteriorated and she was diagnosed with fibromyalgia. The onset of fibromyalgia had brought her life to a halt. She described in great detail the many ways it prevented her from living a full life. When I asked her to tell me more about significant events in her past, however, she got tears in her eyes.

When she was 12 years old, she had been raped by a friend of the family. Twenty years later, she could not remember it without experiencing the horror she felt at the time. As she told me the story, she began to cry, visibly shaking and reliving the event with all of its traumatic emotions. Along with fibromyalgia, Kelly was unmistakably suffering from PTSD.

My new understanding of the role of microglia gave me a different way of putting these separate elements together. How did a car accident, rape, and PTSD build up to a systemic pain disorder?

If my theory was correct, when Kelly was raped as a child, the microglia in her central nervous system became intensely activated. Psychologically, she had tried to put the trauma out of her mind. She told herself she had moved on, but, in fact, she had never gotten over it. On an emotional level, the assault was as upsetting at 32 years old as it had been at 12. At the level of the microglia, their inflammatory response to that trauma may never have completely ended. At the very least, the unresolved trauma had kept the microglia so primed to react that, from the moment she mentioned the event in my office, the full-blown experience of the trauma came rushing back.

When Kelly was 18—just 6 years after she was raped—the microglia in her brain were exposed to another trauma: a car accident with a head injury that directly impacted her brain. Two years after that, she developed widespread chronic pain.

In the past, if an adult complained of chronic pain, it would have been hard to see the relevance of any previous traumas. How different that series of events looked to me now! One assault after another had kept Kelly's body inflamed for the last 20 years. Of course there were serious repercussions.

If, as I suspected, the underlying cause was the upregulation of microglia, a completely different series of events could have had the same repercussions. In another person, might not the tragic loss of a loved one, an infectious disease, and a back injury have brought about yet another disabling illness?

Anything that sufficiently provoked the microglia to create and sustain inflammation in the body had the potential to become a neurodegenerative condition of any sort. The type of assault to the body was less significant than the fact of a chronic inflammatory state in the brain.

When we only address the individual symptoms, the microglia remain hyperreactive. It is only a matter of time before something else—a bug bite, an infection, an accident—sets off the inflammation again.

If Kelly's physical symptoms were ever to improve, we would have to use a comprehensive treatment program to downregulate the microglia. That would include seeing a therapist to resolve the PTSD that was keeping her nervous system inflamed. We could relieve her physical symptoms as we went along, but our ultimate goal would not be to mask the symptoms, but to quiet the inflammation that was causing them. We didn't simply hope to make her fibromyalgia easier to live with. We hoped to cure it.

In virtually all of our patients with chronic pain and psychiatric conditions, the onset of the disease is rarely a singular event. More often, chronic pain evolves as a consequence of a series of assaults on the central nervous system over a period of time.

HOW MANY HITS DOES IT TAKE?

Although Nicole's response to treatment for Lyme and lead poisoning had proven she did not have multiple sclerosis and started her on the road to total recovery, I couldn't help but wonder what had heightened her vulnerability to these assaults. When I took Nicole's medical history, I found the same long series of traumas. The specifics were different, but the story was familiar.

Nicole had developed a smoldering sensitivity to microglial inflammation early on. As a child, she'd had a history of seizures. Although doctors never discovered what was causing them at the time, we now know that seizure activity upregulates microglia and might well have predisposed her brain to inflammation. All injuries, infectious diseases, and toxic poisoning can turn on the microglia.

An avid athlete, Nicole regularly engaged in sports. After a sports injury, she had an operation on her knee. Some days she could walk; some days she couldn't. The problem went on for years and resulted in five operations on one knee, one operation on the other. Because they couldn't find anything else wrong, the doctors decided she must have arthritis. They put Nicole on an NSAID, Celebrex, and told her she would probably have trouble with her knees all her life.

Once we began to calm the inflammation, the symptoms diminished across the board. It was a clear sign that we had shifted the microglia away from their production of inflammatory factors that actively destroyed tissue and into their other role: aiding the reparative processes in the brain.

At their most benign, the purpose of microglia is to keep the nerves healthy, clear up debris, and ensure that the neural pathways are clear. When the body is hit with an assault or infection, the microglia sound the alarm, then seal off the damaged area and start working to limit the damage. Creating inflammation, they form a buffer around the area. They secrete destructive chemicals to kill off and remove the damaged tissue or pathogens in the area, then they summon other cells to help clear away the debris. When the job is done, they resume their more nurturing role, secreting substances that cause the tissues to regenerate, promote neural growth, and initiate repair processes.

Only in a pathological state do they become hyperactive. After too many assaults, infections, injuries, or traumas—whether emotional or physical—they become chronically upregulated, producing inflammatory substances so regularly that they stay "switched on" rather than going back to their role in repairing the body.

Because we do not yet know how to directly "switch off" the microglia, our approach involves peeling back the layers, taking away each thing that is provoking inflammation in the brain. We are working to counteract the cumulative effects of a series of assaults. When we did that with Nicole, the microglia responded. They stopped producing inflammation and resumed their neurological repairs. Clinically, the effect was obvious. Nicole's focus and concentration improved. Her energy started coming back.

How many hits can a person take before getting knocked down? Each of us has a different level of resilience. Some people can take a huge number of blows. Others are born vulnerable and get creamed.

This is where Nicole had an enormous advantage. Temperamentally, she has an extremely optimistic perspective on life. It's her wiring. Despite the devastating experiences of the past few years, she is still finding ways to give the whole thing a positive spin. "Now that I think about it," she says. "It was a helluva good time to drop out. The market stank. They were tearing out the middle lane on the beltway near our house. It's an utter disaster for traffic flow. But I didn't have to drive it!"

Now that she's feeling herself again, she's even managed to come away with some personal insights. "I realize now that my value is not in the work I do, it's in the person I am. Whether my brain works or not, that's not who I am. I'm more than that."

To speed her improvement, Nicole does puzzles in the paper with her husband every day. She goes through brain game books and crossword puzzle books as often as she can. It's impossible to predict whether or not she will regain her former functioning.

It can take a long time for the brain to repair. The process is much slower in older people than in younger people. Nicole is doing everything she can to actively improve her odds. She's started devising tests for herself, to see how well she can handle completing a process. "I take pictures of stuff in my house and sell it on the Internet to see if I will remember to follow through or forget. We make everything into a brain game. My whole life is getting better now."

THE SINGLE POINT OF ORIGIN

Knowing the single point of origin radically changes the way we look at how we get sick, why we stay sick, and how we can recover.

Until now, our best options were to mask the symptoms. Now we know that chronic pain and depression are neuroinflammatory diseases. We have discovered that microglia are the mechanism behind this inflammation. And we are beginning to find ways to address the source of the problem rather than the wide range of symptoms that we had assumed were unrelated.

This knowledge has completely changed the way I practice medicine. My understanding of health and illness is radically different, as a result. By shutting down the inflammation at its source—inside the brain—we can finally have success with diverse and chronic conditions such as fibromyalgia, migraines, osteoarthritis, back pain, neuropathy, depression, post-traumatic stress disorder, anxiety disorders, irritable bowel syndrome, and many more.

In the past, all we could do was evaluate what was happening in the body. Now we know why it's happening.

Chapter 5

HIDDEN CONNECTIONS

HOW ALLERGIES AND MALNUTRITION CREATED PANIC ATTACKS

Nature's slightest deviation from the conduct expected of her is . . . the secret of the best research.

Alan Gregg

At 23 years old, Lindsay Burkett had the job of her dreams. Fresh out of college, she was living on her own in the big city—Washington, DC—and working on Capitol Hill as a congressional aide.

Excited by the privilege, she worked hard. It was her job to remember everything. She was by the senator's side all day long. She went to all of his meetings. She was the one who had to tell the senator the name of everyone who approached him, where they were from, why they were in DC, and what they really wanted to know but weren't asking.

It was like running ahead of a speeding bullet. An excellent memory—heightened by hours of note taking, study, and memorization—was vital to her survival. She needed to review constantly to keep up with all the data, but she had to squeeze in time for that after hours because the days were nonstop. Grueling 12- to 15-hour days were the norm.

With bright young staffers nipping at her heels, she knew she had to be at her best to hold on to her position. Luckily, Lindsay's best was extraordinary. She had always been at the top of her class. But then, so had they. To stay ahead of the pack, she set her sights on "perfect" and ran as fast as she could.

She was always the first to arrive in the mornings and the last to leave. Breakfast meetings with congressional committee members might start at 7:00 a.m. A community event with constituents at the end of the day could easily last long into the night. In between, Lindsay had to summon the energy and brain capacity to brief the senator for back-to-back meetings, often scheduled at 15-minute intervals, while they rushed around Capitol Hill.

If she'd had any time to go to the gym, she would've burned fewer calories than she did at work. The whole culture in DC was in constant motion. There was no such thing as a lunch break. Every activity was laser-focused on a political agenda. Eating for the sake of eating—what would be the point of that?

When she actually started to feel dizzy or couldn't think, Lindsay would try to inconspicuously grab a sandwich from a vendor. Taking the time to eat it felt vaguely self-indulgent. Worse, it was a sign of vulnerability—the last thing she wanted the senator or her colleagues to see.

If any of them knew how close she was to being incapacitated by migraines each day, Lindsay dreaded to think what would happen. If they ever found out she fell into bed at night on the brink of exhaustion, flushed with anxiety, sobbing, and falling to pieces, she'd never work in Washington again.

COMMON MISDIAGNOSES

When she accepted the job, Lindsay knew the migraines were likely to come with her. They'd started in high school when she was 16. She always did well in school, but some mornings, she just couldn't get her brain to work right. It was like a fog was drifting in and out. One moment she was raising her hand in class, eager to answer the teachers' questions, and the next she was struggling to remember what she'd wanted to say.

As soon as the migraines became frequent, her mother started taking her to neurologists. "It's not just migraines. There's some sort of visual distortion going on as well. It makes me feel dizzy," Lindsay explained. A few doctors dismissed these symptoms as common side effects of migraines. Others diagnosed her with vertigo, an inner ear disorder completely unrelated to migraines.

The most promising insight came when she was told she had hypoglycemia. "Your levels aren't all that bad," the doctor told her. "But if you eat more frequent meals and less sugar, it should reduce your dizziness and mental fog." Lindsay adjusted her eating habits on the doctor's advice, and things got better for a while, but then she had an alarming experience on the way to college.

She had always loved to drive. It gave her a satisfying sense of independence and empowerment. When she enrolled in a university that was hundreds of miles away, she looked forward to driving to the campus by herself. After driving all day, the excitement of her arrival seemed to snap her out of a daze. Lindsay suddenly realized that the last thing she remembered was kissing her mother good-bye. She didn't remember driving at all. The implications were terrifying.

She felt a knot of anxiety in her gut that soon became familiar. After that, whenever she got behind the wheel—even for a short distance—Lindsay had to suppress a quiet sense of fear. *What if I get lost in some mental fog and drive off the road?*

It didn't help that this mental fog kept returning all through college. English lit majors are continually writing long papers after reading long books. The ability to concentrate well enough to remember what she'd read—much less think critically—was sometimes nearly impossible. And, of course, the migraines continued.

Wondering if she needed to adjust what she was eating even more, she met with a dietician, who thought her symptoms might be a close match for gluten intolerance. In 2007, no one was really talking about gluten intolerance. Lindsay had never heard of it. When she asked her doctor if she should try to avoid gluten, he told her not to bother. From his point of view, the dizziness, mental fog, and visual auras she described were common in people with migraines. He changed her migraine medication and added antiseizure pills.

Knocking back the migraines with stronger drugs should also eliminate the other symptoms, he said. "Besides, I don't believe in gluten intolerance."

NOT A CRAZY PERSON

By the time she got to Washington, Lindsay was having debilitating migraines that lasted a week at a time. She thinks of that year now as "the migraine period." Powering through, she lived with little sleep, crummy food, and constant stress. If she kept going at all, it was from force of will and heavy meds.

One day, while researching a complicated piece of legislation that the senator was planning to take to the Hill, she felt an odd sense of numbness and tingling in her left arm. Before she knew it, she was short of breath. Her chest felt tight and was getting tighter. In seconds, she couldn't catch her breath. Things started closing in. It felt like the weight of the world was on her chest. *A heart attack? At 23? This cannot be happening!*

As much as she wanted to keep it to herself, she knew she needed help, so she confided in a friend at the office. She tried not to make a big deal out it, but he recognized how serious it was and took her directly to the emergency room. The ER doctor and his nurses rushed her in for a series of tests. When the doctor returned, he was oddly calm, almost smug. "Nothing's wrong with you. You're incredibly healthy. You had a panic attack. Have you ever been diagnosed with an anxiety disorder?"

Lindsay was stunned. Her thoughts were racing. A heart attack would have been frightening and potentially fatal, but some sort of fluke. Now this doctor was saying there was really something wrong with her. As far as she knew, only crazy people had panic attacks. *But I'm not a crazy person. I'm a "perfect" person. I do all kinds of things. How can I be crazy when I'm so . . . efficient?*

When she called her doctor the next day, he sent her to a psychiatrist. It felt embarrassing, but at that point, she was so desperate that she was willing to try anything.

The experience was surreal. When the psychiatrist asked Lindsay what she did as a congressional aide, she ran through an impressive list that included attending hearings, gathering information, tracking issues, answering questions from the media, delivering press releases, drafting documents, making public announcements, and answering some of the thousands of letters and e-mails the senator received every week.

The psychiatrist saw a lot of red flags. "That's a lot for one person to take on! What were you doing just before you had this panic attack? Was something making you nervous? Maybe performance anxiety?" His tone was meant to be compassionate, but to a high achiever like Lindsay, it sounded patronizing and misguided.

"No. You don't understand. I don't get nervous. I was the student speaker at my high school graduation, the president of my sorority in college. I love speaking in public. When the panic attack hit, I was just sitting quietly at my desk, working."

"Have you ever experienced a fear of crowds?"

"No."

"Sometimes it shows up as a feeling of foreboding or loss of control."

"No. I don't have that."

"Do you ever have a fear of being trapped in situations you cannot escape?"

"What?" Lindsay frowned. Where did that come from? "No."

As the psychiatrist ran through the list, a quiet sense of relief came over Lindsay. If these were the characteristics of an anxiety disorder, maybe she had nothing to worry about. These anxieties were so unfamiliar, they almost sounded imaginary. A Gary Larson cartoon flashed through her mind. It described a strange anxiety called luposlipaphobia—the fear of being pursued by timber wolves around a kitchen table while wearing socks on a newly waxed floor.

"I'm not afraid of any of those things. My heart just starts racing. I get shortness of breath, and there's a tightness in my chest—"

As if Lindsay's remarks were irrelevant, the psychiatrist wrote a note on a little white pad. "Let me give you this prescription. I think it'll help."

It didn't seem logical to medicate a condition she clearly didn't seem to have, but Lindsay didn't ever want to feel the way she'd felt that night again. If medication was the answer, so be it.

Curiously enough, the SSRI antidepressant was so soothing that it did make her feel better. "I guess I am crazy then," she shrugged, but she knew she wasn't.

FOOD-INDUCED PANIC

Three years later, Lindsay was still taking the medication and still suffering from inexplicable bouts of anxiety.

The panic attacks and anxiety were genuine, but they produced a strange cognitive dissonance in Lindsay. She continued to insist that she did not have the personality of someone who was prone to anxiety. She was healthy, confident, and well adjusted. She had no history of emotional issues, no family problems, or stress on the job. Her life was great.

It was not clear what was triggering the attacks, but her doctor should have asked what else might be causing those symptoms. Instead, he prescribed an antidepressant to mask the only clues he had for solving the mystery.

But she was about to catch a break.

In Kansas, Lindsay's mother happened to go to a doctor who practiced integrative medicine. Tests showed that she had celiac disease. Since there is a genetic proclivity for celiac disease and her symptoms seemed to fit, Lindsay flew to Kansas City. Her blood tests showed that she did not have the markers for the more destructive celiac disease, but given her symptoms, there was a good chance she did have gluten intolerance. The doctor told her to "try to avoid gluten" and sent her home.

Lindsay started taking gluten out of her diet, but since her local medical doctor didn't accept the diagnosis, she wasn't really sure what else to do. A few months later, her mother sent her an article connecting gluten intolerance with anxiety disorders and migraines. If these connections were correct, then Lindsay's anxiety was brought on by the gluten.

Instead of asking, "What were you *feeling* before the panic attack?" someone should have asked her, "What were you *eating*?" Most likely, the problem wasn't pathological anxiety, it was the sandwich she had eaten for lunch.

According to the article, if someone with gluten intolerance ate a sandwich, it could backlash throughout the body and lead to an inability to concentrate, brain fog, anxiety, even migraines. The article was written by the Kaplan Center, a few minutes away in McLean, Virginia. Lindsay made an appointment immediately.

MEETING LINDSAY

When Lindsay walked into my office, she looked vibrantly healthy. Like many people who work on the Hill, her walk was brisk and determined. She exuded intelligence and an unmistakable aura of confidence that made it easy to believe she was a rising star.

As usual, I interviewed her for well over an hour. After hearing her history and doing an examination, I told Lindsay I was fairly certain that she did not have a psychiatric disorder. The medications, while somewhat helpful, were really only addressing her symptoms and not the cause of her problems. I strongly suspected that her diet might be at the root of her problems. Initially, I recommended a comprehensive treatment plan, including blood and stool testing, acupuncture treatments, as well as craniosacral therapy to address her migraines and neck pain.

When her blood tests came back, the results were startling. Lindsay was extremely deficient in a number of essential vitamins and minerals in her body. Ironically, this bright, up-and-coming congressional aide in one of the richest countries in the world was suffering from malnutrition.

"Of course you're dizzy and can't concentrate," I told her. "Of course your body overreacts to stress. You don't have enough nutrients to support your normal bodily functions. You're severely malnourished."

Lindsay's intolerance of gluten had created an inflammatory state in the lining of her small intestine. No matter what she ate, that inflammation prevented her from absorbing the nutrients.

Food directly affects our nervous systems. If we are eating the wrong things, it can show up in any number of effects: depression, migraines, anxiety, peripheral neuropathy, panic attacks, or pain, among others. The emotional symptoms are not caused by psychological issues, any more than are the physical symptoms caused by an acute injury.

Lindsay was right when she told the psychologist that giving speeches and working in high-stress conditions had not caused her panic attacks. In her case, the cliché was true: It was not what was eating her, it was what she was eating.

If anything, the fact that the inflammation was showing up as anxiety only made her intestinal inflammation worse. To a degree we do not yet understand, our emotions are seated in the gut. We already have strong evidence that emotions affect digestion. In extreme cases, severe stress can damage the lining of the entire gastrointestinal tract enough to cause life-threatening diarrhea.

So Lindsay had been caught in a positive feedback loop. Because she had been eating gluten with undiagnosed gluten intolerance, the lining of her intestines had become inflamed and stopped absorbing nutrients. The inflammation and lack of nutrients had imbalanced her system enough to cause jumpiness, anxiety, then full-blown panic attacks. All of those emotions had damaged the intestinal lining even further.

The medication the psychiatrist had given her and the NSAIDs she was taking to cope with the condition were inadvertently making it worse by increasing her intestinal permeability, which heightened her reaction to gluten, which caused her anxiety attacks.

The good news was, we knew what was happening now. "We will get you through this," I assured her. "We know how to resolve it. We can reduce the inflammation in your intestines and your brain. Then, once you can absorb the nutrients again, we'll replace them. You don't have to worry anymore. We've found the problem."

As she listened to me, Lindsay had tears in her eyes. "Everyone kept telling me I was fine, that it was all in my head! You're the first person to say, 'No. You're unhealthy and here's why.'"

I explained she was suffering from a condition known as leaky gut.

LEAKY GUT

Whenever I mention "leaky gut," most of my patients look at me with a slight sense of alarm, as if they're wondering, "My gut is leaking? What does that even mean?"

Our intuitive understanding of the gut is reflected in our vernacular. We have "gut reactions" to people and situations. When we "know" something deep inside, without knowing how, we say we "feel it in our gut." But other than our discreet trips to the bathroom every day and the ubiquitous pharmaceutical ads about "acid indigestion," what happens in our digestive tract is a mystery to most of us.

And yet, digestive issues are the number two reason people seek medical advice, after the common cold. As many as 60 million to 70 million Americans have digestive diseases—almost half of all adults. How many more must have digestive complaints?

Our digestive tract is made up of a series of hollow organs, linked together in segments like a long, twisting hose compacted inside us. Unwound, it would be 25 to 35 feet long, the height of a two-story building.

Our survival depends on it. None of the food we eat comes in a form our bodies can use for energy and nourishment. We rely on our digestive tracts to convert meat, vegetables, bread, and anything else we ingest into microscopic molecules that can be absorbed into our bloodstreams.

All along the route—from the mouth, down the esophagus, to the stomach, then the small intestine, large intestine (colon), rectum, and anus—the hollow organs are lined with mucosa containing tiny glands that release digestive juices. Every organ along the digestive tract has a layer of muscle to help the food move through the tube. The rippling motion (peristalsis) of muscle movement is like an ocean wave traveling through the organs. One muscle contracts to create a narrow passage, then pushes off, propelling it down the length of the organ, as waves of food and fluid ebb and flow through our bodies.

It begins in our mouths. By chewing our food, we mix it with saliva, which contains enzymes to aid the digestive process. When we swallow, the first major muscle movement takes place. We decide to swallow, but once we start, the process is taken over by the nerves and muscles. The whole process of digestion becomes involuntary.

The food is pushed down to the stomach through the esophagus. A ringlike muscle (the lower esophageal sphincter) at the opening to the stomach relaxes and lets the food in. Stomach acid serves an immune function, killing off many of the harmful viruses and bacteria that might try to invade our body via the foods we eat. It also chemically breaks down our food into smaller molecules that can be absorbed. At the top of the small intestines, juices from the pancreas, liver, and gallbladder mix with our food to further process the nutrients. Muscles lining the digestive tract continually push the partially digested food into and through the intestine.

The "small" intestine continues the process, absorbing most of the nutrients, but, at 15 to 20 feet long, the small intestine is not especially small. Spread out flat, it would cover the surface of a regulation tennis court. In our bodies, of course, it is folded repeatedly to fit into a small space.

Inside the mucosal lining of these folds lies the secret to our ability to absorb nutrients. Tiny projections (villi) aided by even more microscopic projections (microvilli) absorb the vitamins, minerals, and other nutrients from our food, making it available to our bloodstream, where it spreads throughout our body to feed and nourish us. Waste products that could not be used, such as undigested food, are pushed into the colon and eventually expelled in those discreet trips to the restroom.[1]

Allowing us to harvest nutrients from what we eat is such a vital function that it has been easy to assume that the processing and elimination of food was the primary activity of our digestive system. As we are only just beginning to discover, our gut does a lot more than that. As Emeran Mayer, MD, professor of physiology, psychiatry, and biobehavioral sciences at UCLA, points out, "The system is way too complicated to have evolved only to make sure things move out of your colon. A big part of our emotions are probably influenced by the nerves in our gut."[2]

GUT FEELINGS

We now know that our intestinal tract has 100 million nerves—more than our spinal cords or peripheral nervous systems. With this radically new understanding, scientists have tentatively begun to refer to it as the body's second brain.

As Michael Gershon, MD, explains in his book *The Second Brain*, the intestinal tract is far more independent than anyone had realized. It is even equipped with its own senses and reflexes.[3]

Surprisingly enough, our digestive systems manufacture just as many neurotransmitters as our brains. With the advent of "designer drugs"—such as selective serotonin reuptake inhibitors (SSRIs)—we have come to think of depression, anxiety, and insomnia in relation to the amount of serotonin circulating in the brain. Only recently has it become apparent that 95 percent of the body's serotonin is manufactured not in the brain, but in the gut.[4]

Now it makes sense that the side effects of SSRIs often include intestinal problems.[5]

In America more than two million people have irritable bowel syndrome (IBS), which may be caused, in part, from too much serotonin in the intestinal tract. As Adam Hadhazy points out in *Scientific American*, this means IBS—like other diseases caused by an imbalance of neurotransmitters in the gut—could almost be considered "mental illnesses" of the second brain.[6]

IBS may also signal an inflammatory process in the spinal cord or brain itself. An emergent theory on the cause of IBS is that it is a form of central sensitization. Inflammation in the spine increases sensitivity of the nerves controlling the muscles that line the intestinal tract and ensure the smooth flow of food throughout our digestive system. When the nerve signals from the spinal cord and brain to the intestines are disrupted, it can cause the intestinal muscles to spasm, resulting in pain and cramping. The muscles respond by becoming overactive (diarrhea) or underactive (constipation).

As researchers have turned their attention to serotonin levels in the gut instead of in the brain, it has led to even more surprises. In a study of rodents at Columbia University Medical Center, scientists found that when they gave rodents with osteoporosis a drug that inhibited the release of serotonin in the gut, the disease disappeared. Gerard Karsenty, MD, lead author of the study and chair of the Department of Genetics and Development at Columbia, admitted, "It was totally unexpected that the gut would regulate bone mass to the extent that one could use this regulation to cure—at least in rodents—osteoporosis."[7]

Dr. Gershon says, "We have never systematically looked at [the intestinal tract] in relating lesions in it to diseases like we have for the [central nervous system]."[8] Once we have had time to investigate the implications of the second brain, important connections to diseases will be linked to the state of our gut.

We know that problems in the intestinal tract can go much further than heartburn and indigestion or constipation. Crohn's disease, IBS, and ulcerative colitis also arise from imbalances in the gut.[9] Early studies have suggested that imbalances in intestinal bacteria can cause "arthritis, diarrhea, autoimmune illness, B_{12} deficiency, chronic fatigue syndrome, cystic acne, colon and breast cancer, eczema, food allergy or sensitivity, inflammatory bowel disease, irritable bowel syndrome, psoriasis, and steatorrhea." None of these conditions were previously recognized as being related to gut bacteria.[10]

Gradually, physicians reading the latest research are becoming aware that migraines are frequently triggered by food sensitivities that inflame the gut.[11]

Diseases like chronic fatigue syndrome, asthma, and fibromyalgia have a significant relationship to the intestinal tract. When balance is restored, the symptoms are often resolved. Any improvement in the health of our intestinal tract increases the effectiveness of our immune systems.

The question currently being investigated by researchers is: Can we analyze the stool to create a map of all the different types and amounts of bacteria in the gut and use it to predict illness? We're hoping it can be done.

If we have a better understanding of the bacterial DNA, we'll have a much deeper understanding of disease. Bacteria turn DNA on and off.

Celiac disease is not caused simply by a genetic proclivity and exposure to gluten. If it were, everyone with a genetic proclivity would have it, and they don't.

Although 35 percent of the population is genetically at risk for celiac, only 3 percent of that population ever develops the disease. So there is a missing element. Something else happens to set it up. One of the things that seems to trigger celiac is an episode or episodes of infectious gastroenteritis, leading to disruption in gut permeability, but there may be others.

Lindsay's mother had full-blown celiac disease. Considering the fact that Lindsay's genetic risk of celiac was 16 times higher than the normal population, she was lucky when the tests showed she didn't have it. Although her body was having a reaction (making antibodies) to most of the components of wheat, the levels were not high enough to meet the criteria for celiac. In other words, her immune system was cranked up, but it hadn't triggered celiac. We began to calm down her system and remove the stimuli to prevent her from getting celiac, which could potentially cascade into other autoimmune diseases.

HIDDEN IMMUNE SYSTEM

When scientists realized that 70 percent of our immune system was located in and around our digestive systems, it was a staggering discovery. Unlikely as it seems, one of the primary reasons for this is bugs. We are only just beginning to comprehend how much we rely on these colonies of microscopic bacteria. Our health is dependent on the trillions of bacteria in our guts.

Ever since 1674, when Dutch scientist Anton van Loeuwenhoek first observed bacteria with a single-lens microscope, some of our biggest medical breakthroughs have involved getting rid of bacteria. The process of pasteurization, discovered by Louis Pasteur, was based on killing bacteria by heating milk to make it safer to consume. In 1905, Robert Koch won the Nobel Prize for proving that bacteria can cause disease, reinforcing the idea that bacteria are best avoided.

It has long been suspected that the bubonic plague (the Black Death), which wiped out an estimated one-third of Europe's population from the 14th to 18th centuries, was caused by an infectious bacteria. Only as recently as November 2012 did anthropologists finally confirm that this devastating disease had indeed been caused by bacteria, after carefully examining the DNA of skeletons buried in "plague pits" throughout France, Italy, Germany, and the Netherlands.[12]

Although they hadn't known how the plague was being passed from person to person, physicians like Nostradamus, who recommended hand washing and clean linens (free from plague bacteria), earned their reputations by reducing the spread of the disease.[13]

It's stories like this that have led us to, rightly, associate bacteria with disease. By the 21st century, we've established a trend for keeping our environments as clean as possible, improving sanitation, dispensing vaccinations, taking antibiotics at the least sign of infection, and supporting a thriving industry in antibacterial soaps and cleaners.

Our enthusiasm for cleanliness may have taken us too far. We didn't understand the nature of bacterial flora in our intestines and how vital they were to our health. The contemporary "hygiene hypothesis" suggests that it is the continual exposure to bacteria in early childhood that helps us build strong immune systems. When children are protected from contaminants, they are actually at greater risk for asthma, allergies, food sensitivities, and immune disorders.[14]

BACTERIA IN THE GUT

There are 10 times more bacteria in our intestinal tract than cells in our body. Within our digestive system, there are 100 trillion (100,000,000,000,000) bacteria. Among those trillions are 400 to 500 different types, but only 20 types of bacteria make up 75 percent of the grand total.[15]

While we're used to thinking of bacteria as the agents of devastating diseases, their other abilities may be unexpected.

- **Bacteria ward off infection.** A 1988 report by the U.S. surgeon general announced: "Normal microbial flora provide a passive mechanism to prevent infection."

- **Bacteria produce vitamins.** The B-complex vitamins—biotin, thiamine (B_1), riboflavin (B_2), niacin (B_3), pantothenic acid (B_5), pyridoxine (B_6), cobalamin (B_{12})—along with folic acid and vitamin K are produced by bacteria in the gut.
- **Bacteria improve nutrient absorption.** *Lactobacillus acidophilus* and bifidobacteria are bacteria that improve our ability to absorb calcium, copper, iron, magnesium, and manganese, among other vitamins and minerals.
- **Bacteria help fight food poisoning.** In 1993, the Centers for Disease Control reported 20 million to 40 million cases of food poisoning. The FDA estimated the number to be even higher: 80 million. A healthy gut, teaming with bacteria, can help counteract the effects of food poisoning.[16]
- **Bacteria manufacture antibiotics.** Acidophilin, an antibiotic that fights off streptococcus and staph infections, is produced by acidophilus.[17]

On the other hand, bacteria learn. After years of our ingesting antibiotics, pain pills, and NSAIDs that kill them off, these colonies of microscopic creatures are beginning to defend themselves. They have learned which antibiotics to expect and, if need be, they undergo rapid mutations to compensate. Already there are antibiotic-resistant strains of strep, gonorrhea, staph, and tuberculosis around the world.

Harmful bacteria, in some people, have adapted by literally removing their cell walls, in order to move through our bodies unimpeded. When they are exposed to certain antibiotics, bacteria respond by turning on specific genes that create a more hospitable environment for the bugs. They may be microscopic, but they are living organisms. When one of their strategies meets with success, they transmit the information to other strains of resistant bacteria.

Every year, 40,000 North Americans die from infections that no longer respond to antibiotics. Dr. Elizabeth Lipski, author of *Digestive Wellness*, rightly states, "If microbes are becoming more resistant and virulent, we must increase our own resistance and strength to outsmart them. We must boost immune function so that people will be less receptive to infection."[18]

GUT INTEGRITY

One of the best ways to boost immunity is to improve the integrity of the gut. This can be achieved by adding live probiotics, when tests show they are needed. Avoiding things that cause leaky gut—like stress, toxic chemicals, poor nutrition, processed food, food additives, sugar, restructured fats, contraceptives, surgery, antibiotics, pain pills—is also vitally important.[19]

The typical American diet is desperately low on nutrients in the first place. The CDC surveys show that we are eating even fewer vegetables and fruits than we were 10 years ago. Not a single state in the Union had 50 percent of residents who were averaging two pieces of fruit a day. No state had 33 percent of residents who were eating three servings of vegetables a day.[20]

Poor food choices contribute to an imbalance of both probiotics and pH in the gut. When we don't eat enough fiber, the entire digestive process slows down. Without fiber to move things along, the by-products of digestion can concentrate and become toxic, irritating the gut mucosa.[21]

As Dr. Lipski points out, "Even foods we normally think of as healthful can be irritating to the gut lining. Milk, an American staple, can be highly irritating to people with lactose intolerance." Gluten and other food allergens have a similar effect. Steroid drugs can feed fungi in the body and damage the mucosal lining.[22]

NSAIDs simultaneously reduce pain and prevent healing. The lining of the intestines is repaired and replaced every 3 to 5 days. NSAIDs dangerously interrupt and block that process. Once the intestinal tract has been damaged, free radicals are often produced in quantities too large for the body to process. This causes inflammation and irritation, which exacerbate a leaky gut.[23]

The tiny villi in the mucosal wall of our intestines not only allow nutrients to move into our bloodstreams, but they also prevent the absorption of toxins. When the villi are damaged, they lose the ability to discern between nutrients and toxins. As a result, they inadvertently allow toxins, microbes, undigested food, waste, or larger-than-normal macromolecules to leak through an abnormally permeable gut wall.

These substances can affect the body directly or initiate an immune reaction.[24] We call this intestinal permeability (aka leaky gut).

According to Alessio Fasano, MD, one of the leading experts on celiac disease, when leaky gut became known, some doctors were too eager to identify it "as a possible mechanism leading to many problems. The problem, though, is that most of these statements were not based on factual evidence, to the point in which we went to the extreme to develop an entire field called leaky gut syndrome that had very few facts and a lot of fantasies, and that's the reason why the traditional medicine establishment has been so skeptical for many years."[25]

Today PubMed lists nearly 5,000 articles on intestinal permeability.[26] The term *leaky gut* may be associated with the former controversy, but it also offers a vivid representation of the process at work.

WHAT GLUTEN DOES

Leaky gut has been implicated in the growing number of food and environmental sensitivities affecting almost 25 percent of American adults. These are not food allergies, but delayed hypersensitivity reactions.[27]

As many as 40 percent of Americans are sensitive to gluten. One in 100 of those has a severe reaction in the form of an autoimmune disease, celiac disease.[28]

"Imagine gluten ingestion on a spectrum," Dr. Fasano says. "At one end, you have people with celiac disease, who cannot tolerate one crumb of gluten in their diet. At the other end, you have the lucky people who can eat pizza, beer, pasta, and cookies and have no ill effects whatsoever. In the middle, there is this murky area of gluten reactions, including gluten sensitivity or intolerance. This is where we are looking for answers."[29]

Most doctors don't know the difference. Some are unaware that gluten sensitivity can genuinely contribute to hundreds of diseases and that the symptoms may not manifest in the gut, but in other parts of the body.[30]

Years ago, we believed that celiac disease was a rare childhood syndrome.

Today the average age of diagnosis is in individuals between ages 40 and 60. Celiac disease affects more than 2 million Americans—1 in 133 people.[31] Researchers have already confirmed that the dramatic rise in figures is not due to greater awareness. By testing old blood samples, they have shown that, in the last 50 years, the rate of celiac disease has increased fourfold.

Gluten intolerance is now estimated to affect 6 to 9 percent of the American population. Furthermore, people in their seventies, who have eaten gluten without problems their entire lives, are now experiencing gluten sensitivity.[32]

Unfortunately, gluten intolerance is sometimes viewed with skepticism. When the tests come back negative for celiac disease, many doctors dismiss their patients' complaints rather than investigating further. Part of the problem is that, like allergy tests, gluten intolerance tests are not consistently reliable. While gluten intolerance is not an allergy to gluten, we have not yet found a definitive means of identifying it in the blood.

The only absolute way to determine gluten intolerance is to completely remove gluten from the diet for 6 weeks and see if the symptoms improve. It can be hard to tell. If there are other food intolerances and nutritional deficiencies at play, removing gluten may only eliminate some of the symptoms.

Peter Green, MD, director of the Celiac Disease Center, estimates that research into gluten intolerance is about 30 years behind celiac research.[33] Without better research, patients are too often told it's "all in their heads." With a burgeoning series of product lines of gluten-free foods, estimated at $2.6 billion in sales last year alone, it is easy to assume that gluten intolerance is nothing more than a fad.[34]

It's widely known that agricultural changes in wheat production over the past decades have altered wheat significantly and raised both its protein and gluten content.[35] Some ascribe gluten sensitivity to the increase in our consumption of wheat. Gluten can now be found in everything from bread and canned goods to hand lotion and makeup.[36] But the evidence is inconsistent. And the cause may lie in the bacteria in the gut itself. We're beginning to suspect that gut bacteria determine whether the immune system treats gluten as food or as a deadly invader.[37]

In his studies of celiac disease, Dr. Fasano made an important discovery. He studied 47 newborns who were genetically at-risk for developing celiac disease. By the time they were 2 years old, these children had a fairly impoverished and unstable community of intestinal bacteria.[38] As he continued to monitor their bacterial levels, the levels of lactobacilli declined in two children. Both developed autoimmune diseases. One got celiac disease, and the other type 1 diabetes (which has a genetic proclivity similar to that of celiac disease).[39]

Dr. Fasano and his colleagues were excited. "Imagine what would be the unbelievable consequences of this finding," he said. "Keep the lactobacilli high enough in the guts of these kids, and you prevent autoimmunity."[40]

The questions is, was it the chicken or the egg? Which came first, the imbalance of bacteria or the autoimmune disease? Some studies show that intestinal inflammation accommodates bacteria that keep the inflammation going.[41] As we've already observed, bacteria learn and fight hard to survive.

It's a living system, where different choices can be made at any stage. Our genetics help determine our bacteria, but the bacteria can change us—turning genes off and on, adapting as they go. According to Bana Jabri, director of research at the University of Chicago Celiac Disease Center, even if the chicken comes first, the egg can contribute. "You have the same endpoint," she says, "but how you get there may be variable." Such complexity both confounds notions of one-way causality and suggests different paths to the same disease.[42]

DIAGNOSIS

When I saw the test results for Lindsay, her intestinal levels of lactobacilli were so low, they were indiscernible.

When there is disruption in the intestinal tract, we can be sure to find poor absorption of nutrients and general malaise. Malaise is a result of the microglia being upregulated. Everything on the list was an echo of what I now understood to be microglial activation.

Lindsay had presented me with a long list of symptoms: migraines,

PMS, anxiety, panic attacks, pain in her neck and back, and acid reflux. My test results revealed that the real list of problems went on even longer, with one thing stacked on the other:

- Low vitamin D
- Extremely low magnesium
- Musculoskeletal problems
- Severe gluten intolerance
- Irritable bowel syndrome
- Dysmenorrhea

We began to unlayer it bit by bit, asking: What were the pain generators? What else could be contributing to this?

Disease is an evolutionary process. When symptoms are dismissed, ignored, or only partially addressed, the underlying problems steadily worsen. The failure to cure one problem stacks the deck for the next one.

CLEAN BILL OF HEALTH

We treat long lists of problems like Lindsay's in layers, too. One by one, we eliminated the things that were exacerbating her condition until we got results.

For the rest of that year, Lindsay came to the Kaplan Center once every 2 to 4 weeks for intravenous magnesium to address her deficiency in magnesium, and vitamin C to help reduce her oxidative load and repair her cells. We treated her with acupuncture to help reduce inflammation, eliminate her migraines, and rebalance her system to quell her anxiety. We also did craniosacral work to restore motion and flow of the cerebral spinal fluid and relax the fibrous structures that support the brain. This also helped with her migraines. We recommended supplements for her to take at home. To improve her health, she took up Pilates and yoga.

On the Internet, it is easy to find testimonials of people who claim their lives have been changed after giving up gluten for 2 weeks. With Lindsay, as with most people, it took longer.

After 6 months, she started to feel significantly better. Her migraines were greatly reduced. We were slowly weaning her off the strong anxiety and antiseizure medications she had been taking. It took almost a year to get her safely off those drugs.

After 18 months, she came into my office grinning. It was the only time since high school that she hadn't had a migraine. She said she could tell her thoughts were sharper, more reliable. There were no more struggles with brain fog.

During that time, she even fell in love and got married. At the wedding, there was a regular wedding cake and a cake that was gluten-free. She had a little of both, and it was her only taste of gluten in 2 years. At home, she and her new husband even keep separate toasters, to avoid the risk of cross-contamination with gluten. As an extra precaution, she avoids dairy, since there is a strong tendency for lactose intolerance in people who are gluten intolerant. She gave up coffee in the mornings, too. Caffeine irritates an already irritated nervous system and the intestinal tract, so it's counterproductive when you're trying to calm the system.

Lindsay's schedule intensified when the senator she'd been working with asked her to join him on his presidential campaign. She jumped at the chance, but knew it would require being on the go 24 hours a day, sleeping little, eating on the run, etc. On top of which she worried about migraines, brain fog, and panic attacks.

Always trying to excel, Lindsay tackled the challenge proactively. She learned to cook lean protein ahead of time and steam a lot of vegetables, combining them with quinoa, rice, and corn tortillas.

"I had to learn to cook," Lindsay said. "You can't trust restaurants. You go out one night and ask the waiter if an item on the menu is gluten free. The chef says yes. The next time you ask, a different waiter says, 'Yes, but the sauce has gluten.' So you just don't know. It's safer to do it yourself."

When I saw Lindsay again after 6 months on the road with the presidential campaign, she was on the top of the world. "You've turned my life around," she said. "A few years ago, I could never have done something like that. I was focused, driven. My memory was great. It felt like *me*—

the Lindsay I remembered from my early high school days. This is who I am."

At the time of this writing, she has just given birth to her first child, a beautiful healthy baby boy. With the profound malnourishment she suffered when I met her, she might never have been able to have a healthy child, if she had managed to get pregnant at all. Continuing to bury the problem in strong drugs would have eventually cost Lindsay the life and family she loves.

With leaky gut, the deck has been stacked for years, more often decades. The entire intestinal tract is in an inflammatory state that makes it highly permeable. It compounds food sensitivities and generates others. The motility of the gut is disrupted. Nutritional deficiencies mount.

Yet when we quiet it all down and start restoring the integrity to the gut, the secondary problems recede. In Lindsay's case, the migraines and panic attacks simply went away. And gradually the problem is resolved. Not buried in medications. Resolved.

Lindsay is a great example of the validity of this process. She's a home run.

Chapter 6

CONFLICTING TRUTHS

HOW FOOD, MALARIA, AND A FENDER BENDER LED TO FIBROMYALGIA

Are we too enthralled with the answers these days? Are we afraid of questions, especially those that linger too long?

Stuart Firestein

Jada counted 20 adults. Most perched gingerly on the edges of the white plastic chairs in the community center. A few slumped onto the table in loose-fitting jeans and T-shirts, as if they didn't have the energy to sit upright on their own. Three took the precaution of wearing sunglasses to ward off the glare of the fluorescent lights.

The crisp designer jacket that usually served to enhance Jada Peric's assurance suddenly made her feel defensive, out of place. Offering a courteous smile to no one in particular, she chose the chair closest to the door. If it signaled her reservations, so be it. Most likely, her manner revealed it anyway: She was not the support-group type.

When the others began to talk, she felt an unexpected sense of relief as they described the same mysterious symptoms she'd become intimately familiar with in the past few years: widespread pain, stiffness in muscles and joints, changes in vision, light sensitivity, and severe, intolerable fatigue.

"Sometimes, I just cry," one of them said. "My husband asks me what's wrong, but I can't even say. It's just this horrible, persistent ache."

Nods and murmurs moved through the group like a sympathetic tide.

"What bothers me most," said a woman in black sunglasses, "is the way people look at you as if you're making it out to be worse than it is—as if I enjoy not being able to play with my kids or hold down a job." The others winced and shifted in their chairs. Her words stirred up years of painful memories for all of them. The rising tension was palpable in the room. "Even my pharmacist gave me a skeptical look yesterday. What does he think? I'm just chugging down medications with all these side effects for the fun of it?"

Whenever the tone became too harsh, the leader would intervene in a soothing voice, reminding them that "we are all in this together" and gently nudging the group away from bitterness and toward acceptance. To Jada, it felt like resignation. A staunch opposition rose up inside her, blatantly refusing to resign.

This insidious disease had become more and more insufferable these last few months. Burdened with a painful secret to protect, she was isolated from the people she loved. She dreaded to think what a humiliating position it would put her in if anyone at work knew how much she was struggling to get through every day. Surely, her colleagues at the World Bank would lose confidence in her if they realized she'd been diagnosed with fibromyalgia.

Here was a condition once considered nearly as questionable as a UFO abduction. When the World Health Organization confirmed the diagnosis in 1991, based on the criteria of rheumatologist Frederick Wolfe, doctors across the country started applying the diagnosis helter-skelter to anyone complaining of pain, stiff joints, mood swings, bladder infections, sleep disorders, headaches, and PMS. When he saw how indiscriminately the diagnosis was being used, Dr. Wolfe was appalled. "We thought we had discovered a new physical disease," he said, ruefully. "But it was the Emperor's New Clothes."[1]

In the years since, the debate over fibromyalgia has continued to rage. As many as six million Americans exhibit the symptoms, yet it is one of the most difficult conditions to diagnose.[2] Some doctors wonder whether or not it is a disease at all, which raises an even more serious problem: What qualifies as a disease?

"Nobody has a good definition of what a disease really is," Dr. Wolfe admits. "Everybody recognizes that the pain is real and it's severe and it causes people problems. The question that comes up is diagnosis. To sell drugs, you have to diagnose it. To make it a legitimate disease, that you can study and get grants for, it has to be diagnosed. Insurance companies don't want to pay for pain. They want to pay for a diagnosed disease."[3]

With doctors quibbling over what to call it, patients suffering from *whatever it was* had a completely different agenda. "I wouldn't have cared if my illness had a name," a fibromyalgia patient told Claudia Craig Marek for her book *The First Year*. "I wouldn't have minded that there was no cure. I would have been comforted just to know that there was someone else like me, someone who had strange symptoms no one could explain."[4]

Jada had come to the fibromyalgia group for the same kind of solace, but she was not interested in learning to resign herself to a lifetime of misery. No doubt the leader of the group would have told Jada she was in denial. Most doctors might have agreed. The prevailing assumption was that fibromyalgia could not be cured. The best drugs on the market were only able to make patients 60 percent worse, instead of 80 percent worse.[5] As Jada had discovered, even the support groups with the best of intentions had not emerged to share referrals and solutions, but to help people face the "fact" that they would never be healthy again.

Jada left that day with no intention of ever going back. If anything, the taste of resignation she got that day made her more determined than ever to fight. No matter how "realistic" it might be to simply accept that she would never recover, Jada wasn't willing to take no for an answer.

MORE PROBLEMS THAN SOLUTIONS

With fibromyalgia, it seemed the only thing more uncertain than the diagnosis was the treatment. Marek commonly found doctors treating patients "for symptoms they didn't understand with medications that were not helping."[6]

After seeing her own doctor, Jada had consulted an internist, a pain specialist, and a neurologist, to no avail. The rheumatologist who diagnosed her with fibromyalgia had prescribed pregabalin, an anticonvulsant that was the first medicine approved by the U.S. Food and Drug Administration for the treatment of fibromyalgia.[7] The drug itself has such serious side effects that not all doctors are willing to write the prescription. It can be responsible for blurred vision, confusion, unusual bleeding, muscle pain, serious allergic reactions, severe dizziness, difficulty breathing, suicidal thoughts, and seizures.[8] Since she'd been taking it, Jada was reeling. She couldn't help but wonder which of her problems were caused by the disease and which were caused by the treatment.

In her work at the World Bank, she was often required to speak several different languages to communicate with bankers in member countries around the world. In Africa, she had grown up speaking English and Bantu, but she had only recently become fluent in French and German to improve her career. Once she started taking pregabalin, she found herself struggling for words. Was it the side effect of the drug or the progression of fibromyalgia?

The exhaustion alone was a constant burden. She was desperate for soothing, restorative sleep, yet she tossed and turned all night and woke up after less than 6 hours. Even in the night, the pain in her limbs never went away.

Although she had rarely missed work, it was becoming more common for her to wake in the morning with a profound ache that felt as if it filled up every cell, leaving no room for courage or hope. On days like these, there could be no thought of hiding the pain and soldiering on. She was beyond caring. All she could do, as the hours slowed to a crawl, was wait for the treacherous misery to pass.

Year after year, as her condition worsened, Jada's anxiety gave way to a deep, private despair. As she watched her life slipping away from her, she felt a magnitude of emotional devastation she'd never known before. When she sought out a psychiatrist for help, he prescribed

Cymbalta, a serotonin and norepinephrine reuptake inhibitor for depression. The drugs helped reduce her pain and depression. Her headaches and migraines lessened, but the irritable bowel syndrome (IBS) continued. And some days the pain was so overwhelming, she was unable to get out of bed.

With regular days of pain and despair, Jada knew she had only found a partial solution at best. She had no choice but to continue looking for answers.

MEETING JADA

When she heard about the Kaplan Center, Jada found it appealing that I was willing to discuss the complexities of her situation as long as necessary, rather than rushing her in and out of the office, as other doctors had.

In her case, there was a clear trail to follow. Her parents worked for the United Nations Refugee Agency, and the family had lived in Africa while she was growing up. When she was 11 years old, she had a bad bout of malaria. At 14, she contracted amoebic dysentery. The local doctors treated her correctly, but she'd had intestinal complaints ever since. Episodic diarrhea, bloating, and gas were commonplace for Jada by the time I saw her.

When Jada was 16, her parents transferred to Washington, DC, where she attended high school and college. She had always had PMS, but so had most of her girlfriends. It was not until she was back in the States that she started to develop migraines as well.

Eager to return to Africa, Jada joined the Peace Corps after college and was stationed in Uganda. After 18 months, she contracted malaria again. It wasn't as bad as she remembered, but even after it passed, Jada's energy was never quite the same again. She loved being back on the continent and felt she'd found her life's work. Her enthusiasm couldn't have been greater, yet her energy dwindled more every day. It didn't make sense.

By her midtwenties, Jada's body was already stumbling in its attempts to keep her healthy, but no one was connecting the dots. One doctor diagnosed her with IBS, which is not an autoimmune inflammatory bowel disease like ulcerative colitis or Crohn's disease, but rather it is regarded as a "functional" disease, a polite way of saying it's caused by stress. It frequently starts after a gastrointestinal infection that lingers. Whatever caused it, the bloating, gas, and bouts of abdominal pain—not to mention her low energy, migraines, and brutal PMS—were significantly disrupting Jada's life.

Rather than pursue an extended stay in Africa, Jada returned to Washington after completing her 2-year commitment in the Peace Corps. She took a job as a microfinance specialist at the World Bank. Physically, she was not in good shape, but she had grown accustomed to pushing her way through each day by sheer willpower.

Then one day she was carpooling with a colleague when a driver in an SUV ran into the back of their car. It was basically a fender bender. There was not too much damage to the car. But for a body whose health was already teetering on the brink, the jolt was significant. Jada was in the passenger seat with a seatbelt on and came away with a painful case of whiplash.

It was too much. Her body couldn't take it. In the days following the accident, she started getting chronic daily headaches and neck pain. The pain escalated like a raging brush fire, bursting out in unexpected places with little provocation. All of these hits had finally built up to a full-blown case of fibromyalgia. At barely 35 years old, Jada was in constant, debilitating pain.

Few doctors would have recognized the car accident as the tipping point in a long series of assaults on Jada's body. Connecting what seems like a series of individual pieces is still a new concept. They would not have realized that her multiple illnesses were cumulative.

Many would still argue that these were all separate and unrelated events. The science is telling us otherwise. It confirms that chronic pain and fibromyalgia in particular are cumulative, progressive phenomena. More important, when I apply that perspective in my practice, patients get better, after they have not been helped by fragmented treatments.

KNOWING WHAT TO LOOK FOR

It was a classic setup. Malaria had upregulated the microglia in Jada's brain by the time she was 11. Malaria is accompanied by long bouts of extremely high fever. As I now knew, microglia would have provoked that fever in the central nervous system in an attempt to fight off the infection. The malaria episodes ran their course, but they could very well have left the microglia in a hyperreactive state.

When she became infected with amoebic dysentery at 14, it never fully left. In a state of imbalance, her intestinal tract was hypersensitive. It is not uncommon for IBS to develop after a significant gastroenteritis. The IBS complicated her situation because now her digestive process was disrupted, resulting in leaky gut—creating nutritional deficiencies and worsening the inflammation in her body. In this state, it was possible that she had developed food intolerances. If so, the food she was eating was keeping her sick.

By then, her microglia were so easily triggered that she started to develop migraines. Untreated, that inflammatory state was already showing up as anxiety and PMS when she contracted malaria a second time. The inflammation was building. It was not going away. The microglia remember.

If we had known what we were looking at in those days, doctors would not have seen Jada as a healthy young woman. They would have seen WARNING SIGNS like big, red flashing lights. She was already in a very precarious state when she got into the car accident. That trauma was the tipping point that pushed her over into the mysterious, whole body pain known as fibromyalgia.

After our initial consultation, I ran a series of lab tests to evaluate her current state. When the tests came back, they showed that Jada had extremely high levels of antibodies to gluten.

Every time she ate a piece of bread, took a vitamin with gluten ingredients, or exposed herself to secondhand gluten in any way, Jada's microglia reacted with radical inflammation. No wonder she was having so many symptoms. Her body had virtually been screaming to get the message across—with one raging symptom after another—but without understanding the connection to microglia, we couldn't interpret it.

All of those years of eating gluten, not knowing she had a severe sensitivity, had wreaked havoc with the lining of her intestinal tract. The test results revealed it was overrun with the wrong kind of bacteria. She had only negligible lactobacillus. These probiotics are essential to breaking down food and transporting nutrients into the bloodstream.

With so much going on, it was no surprise that she was in chronic pain. By conventional measures, she had a complicated pain condition that no one really knew how to treat.

OUR HUMAN ECOSYSTEM

Most people, even physicians, are daunted by the level of complexity that is required to look at the whole body to find the connections and tie up every loose end.

In fact, the beautiful complexity of our bodies is the reason we're able to thrive. It's astonishing how adaptable we are at the deepest physiological level. Think about how many ways Jada's body found to cope with a series of assaults—infections, emotional turmoil, car accidents, near misses. Every time the microglia were triggered, they turned on inflammation like a toggle switch, but its expression was multifaceted and unique.

Not everyone who gets malaria twice in their lives develops migraines. Many people who have car accidents or amoebic dysentery recover without incident. Our genetic proclivities, our life experiences, our temperaments, and our responses to those experiences all contribute to the teaming ecosystem of our individual bodies.

A fascinating 2011 study by researchers at the University of Madrid points out that all multicellular beings are ecosystems. We are made up of different kinds of cells that cooperate but also compete for resources. We are colonized by so many bacteria that they outnumber the cells in our bodies, and their activities are linked to more processes in our organisms than we have yet begun to grasp. We are regularly invaded by viruses. Some of them are harmful, even fatal, but others are vital in helping regulate our DNA.[9]

As with the ecosystem of the planet we live on, all of the beings in our bodies' ecosystems are constantly changing. Eventually, "all of the entities that form us have been substituted one or more times. Nevertheless, throughout the process, we continue to be ourselves."[10]

When things start misfiring in a dynamic living system like this, how could the solution possibly be a single pill, a single treatment, a one-shot fix? If we are going to restore an entire ecosystem to balance, we have to look at the totality of what's going on.

Faced with the teeming complexity of the human body, doctors are preternaturally disposed to take a simple handshake approach: Here's a diagnosis. Here's a drug. This works fine with acute trauma, where the problem is a single conspicuous thing. A Band-Aid's great for a skinned knee. But when we, as doctors, are too eager to say, "I've got a pill for that!" we may be masking the very symptoms that could lead us to the source of the problem. It's better to listen for all the nuances—everything the patient can remember, whether they think it's related or not—and then ask ourselves: What's going on?

I recently saw a patient who was having muscle spasms, constipation, allergy attacks, and fatigue. Every time he went to a new doctor, he was given a new pill. He was taking Claritin, Singulair, Flonase, Mucinex D, and steroid inhalants against allergies and sinusitis. Many of the symptoms that bothered him most were side effects from all the medications. All of these drugs were treating the branches and leaves, not the roots. At no time was the fundamental problem being addressed. The only thing he could do in the long run? Get sicker.

ENLISTING THE BODY'S HELP

From my point of view, all of Jada's symptoms were variations on a theme. There were multiple physiological assaults triggering the microglia. We needed to address each one, on the well-informed assumption that they were interrelated.

The beauty is, that when we start addressing these things, they all help fix each other. Microglial memory had made her entire system vulnerable to inflammation that was easily triggered. If we could eliminate the things that were constantly working to undermine her health, the rest of the process would be easier.

Since the psychotherapist was a part of my team, I knew she was using powerful cognitive-behavioral techniques and EMDR to give Jada tools to address her anxiety. As I'd explained to her, anxiety was not only a symptom of microglial inflammation, but also contributed to the elaborate neurophysiological and neuroendocrinological feedback loop that kept the microglia inflamed and made all of her other symptoms worse.

Focusing first on the restoration of her digestive system, I recommended the anti-inflammatory diet that strictly eliminates any and all forms of gluten. The diet is simple, but it works well for so many of my patients. It means eating only brown rice, fish, chicken, fresh fruits, and vegetables. Because it eliminates many allergens and food sensitivities, it can provide patients with a clean slate for a few months to help their inflammation subside. When there is a spastic colon, increased bowel movements, and cramping, it is important to quiet the nervous system to restore normal motility, which in turns helps to reestablish a healthy intestinal ecosystem. This we can accomplish with acupuncture, craniosacral manipulation, Chinese herbs, and medications.

With Jada, stool analysis revealed that she still had a parasitic infestation: an amoeba in her intestinal tract and significant imbalance of the normal flora necessary for proper digestion. I prescribed Flagyl, a nitroimidazole antibiotic, to eliminate the parasites. After she had finished that course of antibiotics, we retested the stool to confirm that the parasites were gone, then treated the bacterial overgrowth with Cipro, a fluoroquinolone antibiotic.

In the course of treating patients with antibiotics, we put them on Therabiotic Complete, a combination of families of live probiotics that includes lactobacillus, *Streptococcus thermophilus,* bifidobacteria and *Saccharomyces boulardii.* Studies have shown that use of live probiotics can prevent the occurrence of more serious bacterial infections in the gut, specifically *Clostridium difficile (C. difficile),* which presents with a very severe diarrheal disease that's tough to find and get rid of.[11] So whenever we use antibiotics, we want to do what we can to prevent that.

Although they're vital for eliminating parasites and bacteria, antibiotics wreak havoc with the intestinal flora, the microorganisms that allow our digestive system to function. So I prescribed a daily dose of live probiotics to help "seal the gut." In Jada's case, we knew for certain that she was lacking in probiotics, so it was even more important to repopulate the essential bacteria in her gut.[12]

MAGNESIUM IV

Given her combination of IBS, migraines, PMS, muscular pain, and sleep disturbance, I suspected that Jada was also suffering from a significant magnesium deficiency and ordered a test from our lab. Magnesium is the fourth-most abundant mineral in the body.[13] Good health is impossible without it. It is pivotal in more than 300 biochemical reactions. It supports our immune systems and maintains healthy nerve and muscle function.[14] When a patient has a leaky gut, the ability of the intestines to absorb nutrients is directly affected.

According to the USDA, most Americans (57 percent) do not even get the low Recommended Dietary Allowance (RDA) of 80 milligrams magnesium through their diet.[15] The best sources of magnesium in food include leafy greens, dried apricots, avocados, brown rice, wheat bran, almonds, cashews, soybeans, and bananas—not foods that everyone eats on a daily basis.

Magnesium blocks the NMDA receptor, a glutamate receptor in nerve cells. When the receptor is opened, the excitatory neurotransmitter glutamine, the most abundant neurotransmitter in the body, enters the cells and revs them up, making the neurons hyperreactive.

I often prescribe intravenous magnesium for patients in chronic pain to turn this around. Glutamate upregulation will keep them in pain. Counteracting that process with magnesium quiets down the agitating effect of the receptors. In some people, magnesium has a sedative effect. Taken orally, magnesium can create stomach upset and diarrhea, but the primary problem with taking a magnesium pill is bioavailability. Depending on the form of magnesium and the condition of the gut, as little as 30 percent of magnesium is absorbed orally.

Early on, when we were not getting the results we wanted from oral magnesium supplements at the clinic, we began to administer magnesium intravenously. If a patient has had a long-standing magnesium deficiency, the results can be dramatic.

When Jada's test results came back, her deficiency in magnesium was apparent. Understandably, it made her more susceptible to chronic pain and headaches. A number of our patients have eliminated headaches entirely by correcting a magnesium deficiency. Because of the blood loss during their menstrual cycles, women are more prone to magnesium deficiencies than men. Curiously enough, several women who have been treated with an IV to restore their magnesium were able to get pregnant after trying unsuccessfully for years.

The key to identifying magnesium deficiency lies in knowing what to test. Most doctors assess magnesium by measuring the serum levels in the blood. This is a waste of time. Sixty percent of the magnesium in the body is in the bones. The other 38 percent is predominantly inside the cells of the body's tissues and organs. Only 1 to 2 percent of magnesium can be found in the blood.[16] Cancer patients and hard-core alcoholics living on the street are among the few populations whose magnesium might be so extraordinarily depleted that the magnesium in the blood—the last 1 to 2 percent—might also be low.

While this information about magnesium testing is widely available in the medical literature, busy doctors who remain unaware of it can do a serious disservice to their patients by continuing to test only the blood serum levels of magnesium. If we hope to help patients get better, it's vital that we, as doctors, stay informed about the latest advances in medicine, the important changes in the parameters of tests, and the viability of every test we use at each medical laboratory we rely on.

We run regular quality control evaluations on the practices of our medical laboratories, so we can be sure we're getting information that will do people good. In my experience, it's essential to provide our own oversight. Otherwise, the results we get back can, at best, cost us valuable time by leading us in the wrong direction or, at worst, cause us to prescribe treatments that actually work against the patients' health.

CAN LAB RESULTS BE TRUSTED?

All across the country, more than 200,000 laboratories are certified by the U.S. Department of Health and Human Services to run at least 1,000 laboratory tests. Half the tests are run every day.[17] The reliability of tests is based on four measures: accuracy, precision, sensitivity, and specificity.

Accuracy (trueness) and precision (repeatability) are based on standardized testing methods. In high-quality, certified laboratories, it has long been assumed that these measures are reliable because they are objectively monitored by lab personnel.[18]

Sensitivity and specificity are seen as less reliable, since they are relative evaluations, based on studies found in the medical literature.[19] As new studies come out, some laboratories change the parameters of their tests to reflect the latest thinking, and others don't.

Of course, the best labs try to stay on top of the most cutting-edge research in the major medical journals, but with more than 540 articles published every year in the *Journal of the American Medical Association* alone,[20] it is hard to keep up.

According to the Centers for Disease Control, laboratory "guidelines, standards, policies, and best practice recommendations have typically been independent ventures that serve specific fields or professions." Aware of the problem since 2008, the CDC has recommended a governing body to oversee laboratory medicine and disseminate information about best practices,[21] but in the meantime, there is often a startling inconsistency between laboratory results.

Until I find out which studies a particular laboratory has used to determine the norms for a test, I have no way of knowing whether to rely on the results or not. Suppose a lab result indicates that a patient's vitamin D is "below the normal range." What is that range? Test results don't tell us anything, unless we ask questions.

- **Where did the lab get those numbers?** The lab may be relying on a study from 1995, when a 2009 study established better norms.

- **Who were the subjects?** Maybe healthy people matching the description of the patient were studied, or maybe the norm was based on a completely different demographic.
- **How many subjects were there? 1,000? 20,000?** Sometimes when we do a little digging, we find out that the "normal range" was based on a study of only 150 people in an irrelevant population.
- **What assumptions are these norms based on?** An ELISA test for HIV antibodies, for example, is more than 99 percent accurate, but only if it's done 6 weeks after acquiring the infection.[22] Assuming that the test is valid sooner will yield an inaccurate result.
- **If we treat people based on these results, do they get better?** This is the most important criterion of all.

Before I use any laboratory, my team and I sit down with lab directors and ask questions about how they come up with the values for every test we plan to use. I believe strongly that, as physicians, we have an obligation to find out where they got their numbers. Many of these labs have established their normative values bases on small "idealized" populations.

For years the "healthy" values for vitamin levels have been hotly debated. Up until about 10 years ago, what were considered healthy levels of vitamin D were in fact severely deficient. In 2011 the Institute of Medicine more than doubled the recommendation of daily vitamin D intake. Those recommendations are sure to change, however, because they are based on double-blind controlled studies that are notoriously hard to conduct when looking to define ideal vitamin and trace mineral recommendations. The recommendations also narrowly focused on bone health, and we know that vitamin D deficiency is associated with numerous other health risks.

My local lab lists the lower limit of vitamin B_{12} at 211 picograms/milliliter, yet comes with a footnote stating that more than 10 percent of the population with B_{12} levels below 450 pg/mL may develop neurologic symptoms of B_{12} deficiency. Many of the RDA of vitamins or even what the laboratories report as the normal blood levels cannot be taken as values for health, but for a very marginal avoidance of severe deficiency.

Basing our normative values on a truly healthy population may be a much better idea. But what is healthy? We need to make a careful distinction between what is healthy and what is normal. Considering that the average American is 23 pounds heavier than his or her ideal body weight, is obesity the new normal?

Laboratory values are very powerful. As patients we use these numbers to validate our belief in our sense of health or to confirm illness. As physicians we use these numbers to identify the presence of health or illness and to determine our therapeutic recommendations.

It is critical that we understand what these lab results mean, how the normative values are defined, and what happens if we devise a treatment that shifts the patient to a "normal" value. Does the medicine or procedure make patients better or only change the numbers? If we don't bring a high scientific standard to the process, we will not be able to evaluate the results. Only with rigorous examination, each step of the way, can we build a practical foundation for our medical knowledge in these areas.

USING NEW TREATMENTS WITH CAUTION

Some tests are firmly established—beyond debate—but there is a lot of experimental testing without established values. Too many physicians come back from a conference excited about a new test or treatment, and start recommending it for their patients, without finding out if anything supports its validity besides the company selling it. It's bad medicine. After hearing about a new test or procedure, the next step is investigation.

This may mean investigation of the laboratory procedures or of a treatment proposed for a patient's condition. In complementary and alternative medicine, it is not uncommon to have access to a procedure that has not yet been accepted in mainstream medicine. With integrative medicine, careful evaluation of labs is especially important, since many of the labs are testing for possibilities we are just beginning to explore. The guidelines for these tests are new and unproven.

The prolotherapy that helped relieve Emily's leg and hip pain in Chapter 2 is a prime example. In the 1950s, George Hackett, MD, made the counterintuitive discovery that injecting a slightly irritating liquid into tendon and ligament tissue restored the strength of the tissue. It appears to activate the healing process, potentially even repairing degenerated cartilage or unstable tendons and ligaments.[23] It is now known, more appropriately, as regenerative medicine therapy.

Prolotherapy remains controversial, but more and more studies are beginning to validate the procedure. In the uncontrolled environment of my clinical practice, I have seen hundreds of patients benefit from the procedure, when nothing had helped before. In many cases, years of pain have been relieved with prolotherapy.

When my wife developed hip pain, she underwent arthroscopic surgery to evaluate the joint. Afterward, her surgeon told her she would need a hip replacement. When I asked the surgeon to consider a trial of prolotherapy first, he rejected the idea out of hand, saying it was a waste of time. A good friend of mine at Harvard, David Wang, DO, was doing prolotherapy, so I asked him to treat my wife. After a few months of treatment, her hip pain dramatically improved. Five years later, she is back hiking and fully active with no thoughts of having her hip replaced.

Impressed by the effectiveness of this therapy, I asked Dr. Wang to join my practice. He worked with us for several years before leaving to do research and teaching. I have since done extensive training in prolotherapy.

Although more studies are needed, prolotherapy has shown enough promise that the Mayo Clinic has already suggested that it may be helpful for chronic ligament or tendon pain.[24] Whenever a test or a treatment is controversial, I always initiate a dialogue with my patients, helping them weigh the benefits and risks; then we decide together whether or not to try the treatment in their situation. For a patient with knee pain, for instance, the downside of prolotherapy might be the cost, the pain of the injections, the time involved in weeks of treatment, and the fact that it may not work. The upside would be pain relief and the potential of avoiding a knee replacement. Laparoscopic surgery for knee pain believed to be a consequence of osteoarthritis used to be the accepted standard of care, but has now been shown in two well-controlled studies to be of no more value than a placebo. It doesn't change the condition and may actually hasten the need for a knee replacement.

We discuss the evidence—what we know and don't know—and the limits of the studies. With prolotherapy, there have been more than 45 research reports, but only a few of them were based on randomized clinical trials (the kind of studies that tell us whether the results are due to the procedure or due to hopeful expectations).[25] Other tests and treatments are too new to show up in the literature. So the evaluations fall to us, as doctors.

Most of the patients I see come to me with numerous test results. The problem is not usually that the results are incorrect, but that the right questions have not been asked, so the right tests have not been done. A doctor who suspects someone has diabetes but does not know that 15 percent of people who have type 1 diabetes will also have celiac disease won't bother to test for celiac.

As we discussed in Chapter 5, when Lindsay's doctors diagnosed her anxiety disorder, that was the end of the discussion, despite the fact that she did not have the personality profile of a patient with anxiety disorder. No one asked the most obvious question: Why would she have an anxiety disorder? Her life is good and always has been.

Gluten intolerance, like many allergies, is known to cause anxiety. Yet her doctor asked what had happened to upset her before the attacks, when she should have asked what Lindsay had eaten for lunch. Most symptoms can be caused in a variety of ways. It is preposterous to immediately settle for the most common explanation without even asking about the others.

As I said in the Introduction, doctors are taught that, when they hear hoofbeats, they should think of horses, not zebras. But I'd suggest they would be better off to consider all the possibilities, especially in intractable cases. It may be true that horses are more common, but sometimes it's zebras.

The problem with testing is twofold:

- Knowing what questions to ask to choose the right test
- Knowing the limitations of the test and lab

When patients present with Lyme disease and the doctor orders the standard screening test, called the ELISA test, he needs to know that a high percentage of the results—perhaps as high as 30 percent—are going to show that the patients do not have Lyme when they do (false negatives). The sensitivity of this test is very dependent on when in the course of the infection the test is conducted. Because of this, many physicians switched to the more specific test for Lyme, called the Western Blot, but as it turns out, that test also is prone to false negatives. It isn't as sensitive or specific as we thought, so a number of cases of Lyme disease are likely being missed. In short, we need better tests.

Recently, my team and I heard of a lab that claimed it could measure neuroinflammatory factors and neurotransmitters in urine. Since the literature was telling us that elevated inflammatory factors in cerebral spinal fluid correlated with chronic pain and depression, naturally, we were interested. If someone had found a way to identify those factors in urine, it was a real breakthrough. It would give us an easy way to test for inflammatory factors. A urine sample is easy to collect and doesn't even require needles. For some reason, most people don't like getting spinal taps.

When we contacted the lab, they generously sent people out to make presentations to the study group on several occasions. It sounded promising, to the point that we talked about setting up a small study with the company to evaluate its test.

Before we could get to the study phase, however, both Dr. Michael Lumpkin and Dr. José Apud weighed in. (It helps to have one of the leading physiologists in the country and a prominent psychopharmacologist in your study group.) Looking at the lab reports, Dr. Apud said, "None of this matches what we would expect to see from a test like this. It's in contrast to all the literature. The numbers don't make sense." Dr. Lumpkin agreed.

Neuroinflammatory factors and neurotransmitters can be produced in the brain or in other parts of the body. The only ones relevant to chronic pain and depression were the ones in the brain. That's why all the studies relied on spinal fluid. By the time these factors move from the brain to the urine, they've mixed with neuroinflammatory factors and neurotransmitters from other parts of the body. To create a successful test for urine, the lab would have had to figure out how to identify which factors were produced in the brain alone. They hadn't done that.

Dr. Apud and Dr. Lumpkin knew it as soon as they compared the lab's results on urine to the studies done on spinal fluid. The numbers didn't match.

It was not a valid test, so we abandoned it. Although all of us have busy practices, we have to take the time to investigate, as a matter of policy. If we are going to do cutting-edge medicine, we have to explore options that haven't reached the mainstream yet. But without informed investigation, it's irresponsible to act on the results of a test. We need to ask: What assumptions is it based on? How valid are those assumptions?

The results can be surprising.

WELL-INFORMED DECISIONS

During the flu vaccine shortage in 2008, a study at Walter Reed found that, for women of any age and men between the ages of 18 and 49, half of the standard dose of vaccine was effective. Researchers happily reported that our national supply of flu vaccines would last longer than expected. But the study tacitly made one thing clear: For all of this time, everyone, except men over 50, had been given twice the dose they needed.[26]

Even in the 21st century, when we know so much about the different physiologies of men and women, men continue to be the preferred subjects of drug studies. Whenever laboratories and pharmacies base their recommendations on these studies, the results are inevitably skewed. It has been shown that women's reactions to medications can differ from men's by as much as 40 percent.[27] Yet the laboratory norms are often set for men, and the instructions on most medications continue to recommend different doses for adults and children, instead of for men, women, and children.

Knowing the limitations of the norms does not always give us an accurate alternative, but it does allow us to make adjustments that are better informed. It helps to know, for instance, that the RDA values for nutrients were developed by doctors studying starving adults during World War II. The subjects were very different from our modern population. They suffered from severe deficiency diseases—scurvy, rickets, beriberi, pellagra, kwashiorkor, marasmus—which we rarely encounter today.[28] The RDA for vitamin C was 60 milligrams, the minimum amount needed to prevent scurvy. When we came to realize that vitamin C can provide vital support to the immune system, lower blood pressure, counteract food allergies, help eliminate heavy metals, and inhibit bacterial growth, many doctors began to recommend a 2,000 milligrams daily dose as an optimal healthy intake.[29]

In regard to the RDA, the National Institutes of Health points out that "although the reference values are based on data, the data are often scanty or drawn from studies that had limitations. . . . Thus, scientific judgment is required."[30]

QUESTIONING LAB RESULTS

For my patients, I assume the same judgment is required for all lab results. We have to look at tests that are offered and understand what their quality controls are. It still means paying close attention to the labs to confirm that they match what's going on with the patients.

When we test for biotoxicity, for instance, our local lab sends the samples to National Jewish Health Advanced Diagnostic Laboratories in Denver, since it is one of the leading labs in the country specializing in tests for immune disease.

A few years ago, we started getting test results that didn't match our patients. I called the local lab and said, "I'm not confident I can make clinical decisions based on these tests. The tests were reliable before. What's going on?" The local lab said they had started testing in-house, because they had a better test than National Jewish. When I spoke to the doctors at National Jewish, they naturally insisted their test was more reliable.

Running a test trial was the only way to find out who was right. The local lab agreed to send 20 of our patients' blood work to National Jewish as ordered, but would then run their own test at no cost so we could perform a head-to-head test of the labs. Setting all this up took time. It involved numerous calls back and forth to the various lab directors, reviewing the medical journal literature to confirm the best testing methods, then setting up a system for tracking and correlating the results. But we needed reliable data, so we had to put in the work.

Twenty samples were sent to the local lab and 20 identical samples were sent to National Jewish. We knew we could rely on National Jewish, so we used its results as the standard, meaning National Jewish got 20 results out of 20 right. The local lab got only 2 right out of 20. Since 10 percent is a failing score by any measure, we stopped using the local lab for this test.

The CDC shares our concern. Suspecting that the clinical laboratories were not keeping up with the "continual evolution of medical technology, the emergence of entirely new fields of testing (e.g., pharmacogenomics), and the discovery of new applications for existing laboratory tests," the CDC reviewed laboratory practices across the country in 2007. [31]

Anticipating that lab results were reliable but not up-to-date, the CDC instead discovered that laboratory errors such as these were commonplace:

- Mismatching patients and specimens
- Performing lab tests improperly
- Ordering the incorrect sequence of tests
- Interpreting the results incorrectly
- Communicating the results inaccurately
- Misinterpreting or failing to understand the clinical significance of test results[32]

The labs did not meet the minimum standard criteria for quality, except in cases where clinical guidelines were distinctly provided. The CDC recommended an overhaul of the total laboratory testing processes, where laboratories would be given specific, consistent, and useful testing guidelines from evidence-based medicine—and be held accountable for adhering to those guidelines.[33]

With rigorous statistical analysis, quality control, and extensive oversight, the doctors at the CDC asserted that medical testing would be "an important component in the diagnostic tool kit of a health care provider." But they emphasized that testing was most reliable when used along with other meaningful data and when appropriate questions were asked and answered.[34]

Responsible doctors have to be aware of the limitations of medical testing. Treatment should never be based on a medical test alone. Lab results are only one small piece of the diagnostic puzzle.[35]

KNOWING THE LAB LEVELS

The problem many of our patients face is that they look great on paper.

After extensive tests, they show up in my office at their wit's end—suffering from pain, exhaustion, depression, and severe impairment. Many are still wincing at the memory of doctors who have happily assured them that all their lab results are normal. In most cases, the right tests have not been run, the most current research has not been used to set the norms, or the test they need is not available because we don't know how to do it yet. Either way, the problem is the same: normal labs, sick patient.

When my son, Matt, was a junior in college, his energy plummeted. For a few weeks, he felt sick and was running fevers. The local urgent care center tested him for flu and did a chest x-ray. When both tests were normal, they sent him home. As Matt's condition worsened, he called me. By that time, his fever was 102 and he was having difficulty breathing. I told him to go to the emergency room.

The physician's assistant (PA) in the ER looked at the labs from the urgent care center. When he evaluated Matt, he didn't hear any wheezing; his lungs were "quiet." Before sending Matt home, without a diagnosis, a treatment, or a follow-up plan, he gave me a courtesy call. "It's nothing to worry about. I think it's just a virus."

Based on the conversations I'd been having with Matt over the past several days, I disagreed—he sounded quite sick to me. "Did you do a complete blood count?" I asked. A CBC reveals the white cell count, which might indicate the presence of a bacterial infectious process.

"No."

"How about a peak flow?" A peak expiratory flow rate meter is a small, handheld tube that measures the speed of expiration. Low readings indicate the airways are constricted.

"No."

"Run the count and do the peak flow," I told him. "If the flow is under 400, give him an aerosol treatment and call me back."

His peak flow was even lower than expected—well under 200. Matt's lungs were "quiet" because of bronchospasms of asthma. The aerosol treatment brought Matt's peak flow back up over 400, which significantly improved his breathing, but his white blood count was extremely high.

The PA assured me that as soon as he saw that, he immediately tested Matt for mononucleosis. "The test was positive," he announced. "He's got mono."

Mononucleosis is a benign virus. With a white blood cell count this high, I was concerned that Matt might have acute leukemia. My wife drove 4 hours to the university and brought him home.

I took him to my friend Tom Butler, MD, who is a hematologist, and told him about the mono diagnosis but not my concerns about the possibility of leukemia. He examined Matt and assured us that he most likely had mono. But something bothered him about the lab results. As he looked them over, he muttered to himself, sensing that things were not as simple as they appeared. "Let's do a couple more tests," he said.

He repeated the CBC with a microscopic examination of the blood and, instead of relying on the lab report, he looked at the cells himself. Then he conferred with a colleague in the lab. Both of them deduced that it was probably mononucleosis, not acute leukemia. They did, however, recommend that he be retested early the following week.

The repeat test not only confirmed that Matt did indeed have mono, but also resolved the significant insomnia problem I had recently developed. More than anything, I wanted to hear it was just the flu or mono, but I was also immensely grateful for Dr. Butler's thoughtful and thorough consideration of Matt's condition. This is my son. And I'm all too aware that not knowing the appropriate levels for lab results makes them virtually useless. Laboratories send their results to doctors, not patients, on the assumption that the doctors will know the implications of the results, but that is not always the case.

Since no one person can know the latest thinking about the levels for every test, it's vitally important that we consult with others to expand the base of our knowledge. Otherwise, it can leave our diagnoses in question.

DIAGNOSIS

With our patients, we often have to send out tests to more than one lab. Even reputable labs vary on particular tests. We know exactly which labs to use for which tests, and we regularly check to confirm that their procedures haven't changed.

When we got the results back from the various labs we used for Jada, there were a half dozen issues that might have been upregulating her microglia. The list included:

- Extremely low vitamin D
- Extremely low magnesium
- Gluten intolerance
- Amoebic dysentery
- Bacterial overgrowth
- Sleep disorder

We then began treating her entire body comprehensively, using:

- Manual therapy
- Live probiotics
- Elimination diet
- Magnesium IV
- Prolotherapy
- Chinese herbs

- Physical therapy
- Cognitive-behavioral therapy
- Antibiotic and antiparasitic medications

Acupuncture calmed her nervous system and addressed both her anxiety and ongoing neck pain. Manual therapy alleviated the myofascial component.

In the beginning, Jada came to the clinic once or twice a week, scheduling a few treatments each time, for 6 months. For the first few weeks, she had a magnesium IV each time, then had an appointment with me, the physical therapist, or the psychotherapist afterward.

After weeks without gluten, Jada started to feel better. She was already beginning to function better. She had always resisted the idea that she was doomed to live in pain for the rest of her life, but the prospect still loomed in the back of her mind. Avoiding gluten entirely and supplying her with intravenous nutrients dramatically boosted her body's ability to absorb the nutrition it so desperately needed. Low-dose naltrexone helped soothe the inflammatory response of the microglia. At last, Jada was no longer being sucked into a downward spiral.

Her irritable bowel syndrome resolved within a month. The chronic headaches went away in 4 months. Now, once a year, under exceptionally stressful circumstances, Jada might get a migraine, but it is rare. Overall, the pain she experienced was reduced by 90 percent. Her energy was 80 percent better and continuing to improve. Her ability to focus had returned. She was back at work and doing Pilates and yoga several days a week. Jada's joy in life had returned.

NO LONGER GUESSING

Jada's recovery wasn't based on any one thing, but on a comprehensive approach that allowed us to solve a problem in a complicated human ecosystem. Each of Jada's doctors had focused on one thing, never the whole. They couldn't understand her pain, much less treat it, because they had completely failed to recognize the nature of the problem.

Knowing about microglia gives us the key to the locked door. Instead of guessing at what might be behind it, we can now ask informed questions that we never knew to ask before, pursuing an in-depth investigation into the body's cumulative response to assault. Understanding at last how all these symptoms are related, we can follow the story, see how it evolved, and know what we need to do to intervene.

Now we're treating roots, not branches. Now we can talk about total recovery.

Chapter 7

UNSUSPECTED IMPACT

HOW CHILDHOOD ABUSE AND INFECTION CAUSED CHRONIC PAIN

Interpreting the clue and realizing its possible significance requires knowledge without fixed ideas, imagination, scientific insight, and a habit of contemplating all unexplained observations.

William I. B. Beveridge

Sharing childhood memories was the last thing Sarah Nitti expected when she came to see me about a running injury. As soon as she walked into my office, she handed me a folder of the careful records she had kept. An aspiring physician herself, she anticipated that I'd want to know about her treatments by dozens of specialists in the two increasingly painful years since her IT-band surgery. And, of course, I did, but I also knew that if we had any hope of finding the source of the problem, we'd have to go back further than that—all the way back.

As Sarah told her story, I was listening for a pattern. I wondered why a vibrant, 23-year-old athlete was constantly getting sick and suffering from chronic pain. What had triggered the microglia in the first place? And why had that inflammation never subsided?

To her mind, the real problems had begun when she was 20. While she was training for a 10-mile race, she felt a sharp pain on the outside of her right leg. Because her friends were counting on her, Sarah felt compelled to run the race, so she kept training for 2 more months.

Naturally, the stress and intensity of the race made the pain even worse, but she put up with it. After the race, she stopped running for 3 months. It didn't help. Despite the rest and ice, her leg hurt all day long and all through the night.

By midsummer, she consulted an orthopedic surgeon, who diagnosed iliotibial (IT) band syndrome, a common injury among runners, producing swelling and pain along the band of fascia that runs from the pelvis to the knee. The surgeon gave her a series of cortisone injections that ultimately hurt more than the minimal relief they provided.

With the school year approaching, Sarah told him he would have to find another approach quickly, so he recommended IT band release surgery, which would relieve the pressure by lengthening the IT band. It meant she would have to go back to college on crutches, but it was better than being in pain. At first, it seemed like the surgery had worked.

When she gave up the crutches after 2 weeks, she took it easy walking around campus, and her leg felt fine. So she started to test it—walking more quickly between classes, tentatively cycling, even jogging up a few flights of stairs. To Sarah's surprise, her IT band didn't seem to object.

Encouraged, she picked a brisk, sunny day in November to go for a run. There was a path around the lake she particularly loved. It had been almost 8 months since the race, and memorable moments from the hours she had run along this path came back to her in flashes of nostalgia. She missed the indomitable rhythm of her feet hitting the ground, the solid forward motion, the pounding of her heart, keeping time. *If only I could have that back again . . .*

She left at 6:00 a.m. It was cold at first, maybe 40 degrees, and she was out of training, so it took a little longer to warm up, but 15 minutes in, her legs seemed to come awake—at long last—and remember. Taking the initiative, they shifted into a higher gear on their own. A more confident, powerful stride emerged. She was really running now. And it felt good.

Covered neck-to-toe in Gore-Tex, she picked up speed and started to sweat. It was all coming back. If one of the students hanging out on the grass had taken her photo, she would've been surprised to see she was smiling. With her eyes focused on the distance, all she knew was that she felt more invigorated with every stride.

As she sliced through the chilled autumn air, the thin layer of moisture on her heated face grew cool, refreshing. Everything was working together so beautifully that the first jolt of pain in her leg seemed surreal. *This can't be happening. The pain isn't even in the same place as before!* She tried to keep going, but in her heart, she knew it was over.

Fighting off the urge to sink into self-pity and weep, Sarah took three long, last strides and stopped. She looked at her watch. Thirty minutes. That was it.

MEETING SARAH

Discouraged, Sarah went back to the orthopedic surgeon. "You have to give these things time," he said.

Hiding her disappointment, Sarah stoically told her volleyball club she wasn't ready to come back. She managed to cycle and swim regularly, but any kind of running or jumping at all put her in pain. Every 4 months or so, she'd go back to the path by the lake and try to run again, but in every single instance, it hurt. So she kept doing what the surgeon advised: giving it more time. While she waited, though, her condition got worse. Soon it wasn't just leg pain. It had moved to her hip and lower back.

On our initial meeting, I pressed her for more information. What had her health been like before the injury? What else had happened?

One night in college, she had to be rushed to the emergency room for bronchial spasms. It was frightening to feel like she couldn't breathe. Doctors had diagnosed her with asthma and given her an inhaler to use before exercising, so she knew she was vulnerable to respiratory problems. But lately, she seemed to catch any bug that was going around. Almost once a month, she came down with a cold or the flu.

As if it were something to be ashamed of, she reluctantly confessed her fear that her immune system was failing. She was tired even after a good night's sleep. She ate right and exercised, trying to live a healthy life, yet she was sick all the time.

"What else happened?" I asked, drawing more and more of the story out.

"I don't know if it's relevant," Sarah said, "but in high school, I hurt my back playing volleyball and ended up with two bulging discs between the fourth and fifth lumbar vertebra, as well as the fifth lumbar and first sacral vertebra." She was quick to point out that she'd gotten used to low back pain over the years, but now, for no apparent reason, it seemed to be getting progressively worse. A lot of the time, she had trouble sitting at a desk because of the extreme pain she was in. Every night, she struggled to find a comfortable position in the bed or even on the floor.

From all appearances, she was a smart, optimistic student with a bright future ahead of her. And yet, at 23 years old, she couldn't participate in any of the sports she loved, and she felt increasingly exhausted and in constant pain. The truth was that, by the time Sarah finished college, pain was starting to take over her life. "It doesn't make sense," she said. Above all else, she wanted answers.

Sarah's goal was to be a physician. As part of her preparation, she took a research job at a major medical center working with a mentor who was a physician specializing in myofascial pain. Believing her to be a promising student, he took a keen interest in her health.

When he performed a physical exam, he was startled by the results. Her hip, leg, and back were so sensitized that he characterized her as having as both allodynia and hyperalgesia (a temporary increase in sensitivity to pain that has evolved from another illness or infection). Her mentor kindly offered to treat her without charge.

To address the trigger points, he engaged in multiple dry needling treatments. Usually they are not painful, but in Sarah's hypersensitive state, they were excruciating. The pain would subside briefly but then come back in full force a day or two later. Sarah also received treatment from a physical therapist he recommended, but by then, she was experiencing intense pain in her leg, hip, and back for 2 to 5 days at a time. The treatments reduced her pain dramatically, but ultimately, it always returned. That's when her mentor referred her to me.

My initial physical exam revealed some instability in the medial collateral ligament of Sarah's right knee. Beyond that, her nervous system was so agitated that it gave her an exaggerated flinch response. Her reflexes were so overreactive that it raised the possibility of multiple sclerosis. To find out, I ran a neurological exam, but the results proved she didn't have MS.

With her heightened pain and sensitization, it was possible that she had fibromyalgia. She definitely qualified for part of the diagnosis: pain in all four quadrants of her body for 3 months or more. The remaining criteria relied on the experience of pain in at least 11 of 18 tender points along the neck, chest, shoulder, hip, knee, and elbows.[1] Recently, even more points have been added because Frederick Wolfe and others at the American College of Rheumatology began to recognize that many patients with fewer than 11 tender points still had significant fibromyalgia.[2] Sarah, by contrast, was sensitive at all 18 tender points.

Sarah's mentor had rightly identified her widespread myofascial pain, but I knew that since the pain wouldn't subside—even with treatment there had to be other issues. What could be causing her nonhealing injuries, sickness, and pain? What else was going on?

EVALUATION CHECKLIST

Among a nearly endless number of possibilities, the areas I eliminate first, by clinical evaluation and laboratory testing, are:

- Physical trauma
- Psychological trauma
- Medication side effects
- Infectious diseases
- Celiac disease/gluten intolerance
- Nutritional deficiencies

- Musculoskeletal injuries
- Intestinal/digestive disorders
- Genetic issues
- Environmental toxins
- Hormonal disorders
- Autoimmune diseases
- Sleep disorders

Few conventional doctors would even consider evaluating a patient's overall condition in this way. They do their best to treat the symptom presented to them and try to steer clear of the complexities involved in healing the patient as a whole.

After years of clinical practice, I have found that people suffering from chronic conditions that are not alleviated with conventional medicine alone often have problems in several areas on this list. While we are always exploring new areas and looking for useful biomarkers, each of the items on this long list has a direct physiological link to the regulation of microglia.

Sarah had already told me about a series of physical traumas, including and preceding her original complaint, although I suspected there were more. It was also obvious that she would be resistant to discussing the psychological aspects of her condition, but I was planning to address it before our 2-hour interview was over.

With every patient, it's a matter of layers. In the interview, we gradually uncover layers of physical and emotional assault that have provoked an inflammatory response from the microglia. In the treatment, we select the right order to address the issues, careful not to overwhelm the patient's body or budget as we go. Most of the work we do is covered, to some extent, by insurance, but the amount of coverage will be variable according to each individual's insurance policy.

The next possibility on the list was infectious disease. Because we were in Washington, DC, where Lyme disease is common, I asked if she'd been camping or hiking in the area. In fact, she had gone hiking 3 years earlier. She did not remember being bitten by a tick, but it was a possibility we could test.

ORIGINS OF LYME

Lyme disease has been on the rise since 1991 and today is the most common vector-borne disease in the United States.[3] (Any infectious illness that is transmitted by blood-sucking arthropods—mosquitoes, ticks, fleas, mites, and lice—is vector borne.[4]) In 2011, there were as many as 31,773 cases, concentrated in 13 states in the Northeast and upper Midwest.[5] Around the world, it can be contracted in Europe, Asia, Africa, Australia, and South America. According to the CDC, it is a serious threat to human health. Initially, the symptoms may be mild, but if left untreated, the bacterium *Borrelia burgdorferi* (Bb) can spread to the nervous system and joints.[6] When that happens, it can be devastating.

Back in the 1970s, the children of a small village in New London County, Connecticut, started coming down with a mysterious illness every summer. The swollen, aching joints and feverishness might have been rheumatoid arthritis, except that it behaved like an infectious disease, spreading among the children who liked to play in the woods.

Researchers descended on the town, looking for clues. They tested the local water and air for microbes, but couldn't find the cause. When they questioned the children, some of them said they'd had an itchy skin rash just before their joints started aching. A few remembered being bitten by a tick.

By the mid-1970s, the scientists had enough data to identify a new disease. They named it after the village—Lyme—but they weren't sure what caused it. Not until 1981 did researchers in Montana discover that Lyme disease was transmitted by ticks.[7]

A woman in Surrey removed a tick from her foot one summer and spent the next few weeks fighting off symptoms that felt like the flu. Two years later, she was bitten by another tick. Afterward, a growing sense of fatigue came over her. Her joints were as painful and stiff as if she'd had arthritis. Her doctors assured her she didn't, but it never occurred to them that she could be infected with Lyme disease. Over the next 2 years, her symptoms got progressively worse until she had to leave her job and take early retirement.[8] Sadly enough, it's a familiar story.

The standard treatment for Lyme is a 2- to 4-week course of antibiotics. Yet the CDC admits that up to 20 percent of patients will continue to have lingering symptoms—fatigue, pain, joint or muscle aches—sometimes lasting more than 6 months after treatment.[9] As many as 60 percent of untreated patients will develop arthritis that lasts for years, often settling in the knees.[10] In these cases, tests may show high titers of Bb-specific antibodies and Bb DNA in their joint fluid.[11]

Known as post-treatment Lyme disease syndrome, it is so widespread that numerous trials are currently being conducted at the National Institutes of Health in an attempt to understand it.[12] Some researchers theorize that the initial infection provokes an autoimmune reaction that continues to create serious symptoms long after the antibiotics have killed the bacteria.[13] Others assume that the symptoms linger because of residual damage to the immune system and tissues that took place during the infection.[14]

Even organizations dedicated to the disease rarely see evidence of total recovery. With delayed diagnosis, patients are given a lengthy course of intravenous antibiotics, then can relapse after a variable period of remission. "The length of time a person has been infected before treatment, whether the patient has been given sufficient treatment, and whether there are co-infections present, can all have a big impact on a patient's recovery."[15]

In an effort to call attention to the problem, grassroots organizations around the world have begun to mobilize. In May 2013, a Worldwide Lyme Disease Awareness Protest took place in 28 countries, calling for new testing and education about the disease. The group has urged government health organizations to reexamine the current testing for Lyme, asserting that it fails to identify almost two-thirds of the cases.[16] Unfortunately, in the meantime, a lot of people suffering from the symptoms of Lyme disease go undiagnosed.

SEARCHING FOR PHYSICAL AND EMOTIONAL CLUES

While I tested Sarah for Lyme, I also ran tests to evaluate many of the other items on the list. Taken together, all of the items on the list would reflect her total body burden. She did have trouble sleeping, but it was often associated with back pain rather than other primary sleep issues, such as apnea or restless leg syndrome. I started asking questions about Sarah's more distant past.

"What else happened when you were a child?"

It turned out Sarah had been a gymnast as a child, but for some reason, she repeatedly injured her left ankle. After the third injury, the doctors said she had to quit. She was 10 years old.

At 17, she traumatized her left knee in a basketball injury and couldn't play for an entire season. The doctors didn't see anything on the scans but operated to clean up the debris.

And then there was the dysmenorrhea—cramps that nearly paralyzed her with pain every month. They had started in high school when she was 16 and lasted to this day. The only thing that had ever diminished the pain was heavy narcotics. She didn't like the idea of taking them, so she tried to limit the drugs to the very worst day. On the other days, she would lie in bed and cry from the pain.

Any one of these things would activate the microglia, but I still had questions. With a picture like this, there's always something else going on. If I didn't find it, she wouldn't get better.

THE IMPACT OF GRIEF

When Chloe Jacobs, age 52, developed a painful rash, it was diagnosed as shingles. Her doctor gave her a topical antiviral cream that eliminated the painful rash, but not long afterward, it returned. That was unusual. Shingles doesn't typically come back. Only 24 people out of 10,000 with shingles ever get it again.[17]

Chloe made an appointment with me. As usual, I did a long, attentive interview, asking about her life and her medical history. Even if I hadn't asked, her grief would have been apparent.

A few months before, Mark Benson, the project manager at the advertising agency where she worked, had died unexpectedly. They had worked closely together as a team for 7 years, developing presentations, cultivating new clients, and sharing the ups and downs of a fickle industry. Mark was the kind of man who would be missed in their community, but for Chloe, he had been a supportive friend and confidant. The loss was immeasurable.

His death hit her harder than she expected. And a day after the funeral, she got shingles.

Years ago, when a doctor believed that an emotional issue had caused a physical reaction, he would have called it psychosomatic ("all in her head"). Despite the fact that more than 50 percent of people who suffer from depression also experience pain, pain was not even acknowledged as a symptom of depression until 2013, with the publication of the American Psychiatric Association's *Diagnostic and Statistical Manual of Mental Disorders (DSM-V)*, used by mental health professionals to categorize mental illness.

Understanding the function of microglia took the mystery out of the connection between emotional and physical pain. Chloe's grief had compromised her immune system. Shingles had simply exploited that vulnerability.

After observing the ping-pong effect with Charlie (in Chapter 3), where his depression worsened every time we reduced his pain, and vice versa, it wouldn't surprise me if eliminating shingles the first time had somewhat intensified Chloe's emotional pain. The microglia had been upregulated by her grief. A topical cream was not likely to be enough.

When the shingles recurred, I approached it on three levels at once. Acyclovir, an antiviral medication, treated the rash. Acupuncture relieved the pain and size of the rash. Grief counseling helped alleviate the emotional suffering that was sustaining the underlying state of microglial inflammation.

Two weeks later, the pain and rash were gone and didn't return. In some ways, Chloe was fortunate that her body had immediately signaled that something was wrong. When emotional wounds are long-standing, it can be more difficult to find the connections.

ABUSE CAUSES INFLAMMATION

For Sarah, the trauma of her childhood was the key. In the past, I would have known it was relevant, but would not have known why. Grasping the physiology behind these symptoms led me down a very different path of inquiry. Not only did I ask new questions, but also I had a much deeper understanding of why some of the questions I had been asking all along were relevant. By the time I met Sarah, my thinking process had matured. Now when I asked, "What were things like at home when you were growing up?" I knew the answer was vital—not just to her well-being or recovery, but to her very survival as well.

At Sarah's initial visit, she admitted that her mother had been a raging alcoholic, but she hadn't wanted to discuss it. It took time for us to develop the kind of trusting rapport she rightly needed before she felt she could confide in me. When the story did come out in a burst, it was apparent that all the physical pain she had been describing was just the shining tip of a very ominous iceberg.

"I felt like I was walking on eggshells," Sarah admitted. "My mother was not the type of alcoholic who drank and slept it off. She was angry and emotionally abusive on a daily basis throughout my entire childhood. She told us things that no kids should ever be told, like 'You're a worthless piece of crap!'"

The memory alone made her pale. "When I was 10, she would scream at me, calling me a whore. Basically, she tried to make everyone feel worthless. And in a certain way, it worked. I think it's why I've judged myself so harshly my whole life. If your own mother tells you, for 15 years straight, 'You were a mistake! You should never have been born!' it affects you.

"Of course, I learned to keep my guard up and pretend it didn't bother me. No matter what I was feeling, I wouldn't let it show. Sometimes my friends would tell me I seemed cold. I didn't feel that way inside, but my defenses were so strong, I'm sure it looked that way. It was hard for me to open up. If I had exposed my true feelings in that house, I would never have survived. So I put on a brave face.

"It was a pretty traumatic childhood. A lot of dysfunction. I took on the perfectionist role, trying to be nurturing to everyone else. My oldest brother internalized all the turmoil and was morbidly obese with cardiomyopathy by 29. My middle brother was the angry one, always losing his temper and becoming violent. At home he would fly into rages like our mother, screaming and throwing things. My father's reaction was to tell all of us to leave the room. Avoidance was his only solution.

"My mother had a successful legal practice in town, yet she was repeatedly being hospitalized for broken bones and injuries because she drank so hard she couldn't function. No matter how serious the injury, she would get out of the hospital and drink herself into a stupor again.

"But no one would've ever guessed it. All our family problems were supposed to take place behind closed doors. No one was allowed to talk about it—not at home, much less in public. Home was never a safe place."

Like many children from abusive homes, the very thought of revealing the family secrets to a therapist was anathema. As a teenager, Sarah asked to see a therapist, but her mother absolutely refused, then ridiculed her for "needing help." The best Sarah could do was to move out of the house as soon as possible.

Despite the constant trauma they inflicted, she felt obligated to care for her parents, even though they were in their early sixties. The inexpressible strength of the bonds with her family were, in many ways, taking a toll on her health.

Whether or not Sarah could find a way out, I knew we had to look for a solution. My new understanding of the consequences of long-term microglial inflammation gave my emphasis on the psychological issues a new urgency.

THE HIGH COST OF UNRESOLVED ISSUES

The evidence is in. Depression, chronic anxiety, and PTSD are neuroinflammatory and neurodegenerative. Resolving them is no longer an option. It's not a bid for a happier, more fulfilling life. It's a matter of life or death. If these issues are not resolved, neurodegeneration will be progressive. Disability and incapacity are absolutely certain to follow.

For her entire life, Sarah's very survival had depended on locking the door to the emotional turmoil and abuse of her family life. If I could not persuade her to open that door now, her future was bleak.

The test results would give us important insights into how her underlying trauma was manifesting. But if physical and emotional trauma exist as opposite ends of the same pole, we would have to treat both to make her well. Otherwise, her symptoms would keep pinging from one end of that pole to the other. If we treat depression as one thing and pain as a completely separate symptom, we haven't treated the underlying causes, so she will experience only partial recovery at best.

Depression and pain are extreme outlets for microglial inflammation. There are many other manifestations. When the microglia are creating neuroinflammation, the symptoms may show up first as depression, then pain, then fatigue or anxiety or a backache, but it's all the same: It's inflammation in the brain. If we treated only the physical manifestations of pain, the emotional manifestations would flare up and vice versa. With the microglia inflamed, the pain always reignites, quashing the ability to heal and quite literally hastening degeneration and disability.

DIAGNOSIS

When the tests came back, they revealed that Sarah did not have gluten intolerance or celiac disease. She did have severe hypomagnesemia. In her case, her intracellular levels were low enough to put her at risk of cardiac arrhythmia and sudden death.

As we've seen previously, magnesium prevents too much activation from the nervous system by helping to suppress the NMDA receptor for glutamate (the most abundant and excitatory neurotransmitter in the body). Sarah's heavy, irregular periods had contributed to the problem, leaching magnesium from her body. In her severely deficient state, her nervous system stayed wired. That's what had caused her hyperactivated reflexes and kept her in an agitated state. The radically low magnesium alone would have caused terrible PMS, heavy bleeding, and depression.

She started coming in twice a week for magnesium IVs. Her levels were so low that it took five or six treatments before she noticed a difference, but when she did, there was less pain, better intestinal motility, less PMS, lighter bleeding, and improved energy. At that point, she transitioned to oral magnesium supplements.

Curiously enough, the genetic tests also showed that Sarah had exceptional vulnerability to mold and to toxins acquired from the tick bite. Some people have fewer reserves against the onslaughts of the world. Unable to process the toxins secreted by molds and ticks, their bodies accumulate the toxins. It is often hard for people to fully recover, and we are not yet entirely sure why. We're still missing other pieces of the puzzle; it's an evolving concept.

One way we can observe it is in a patient's genetic sensitivity to environmental biotoxins. Patients with certain genetic patterns appear to lack the ability to break down environmental toxins. The rest of us accomplish this effortlessly. Sometimes the issue is only with mold toxins. Sometimes the problem is with the toxins associated with tick and spider bites. Sometimes it's both. We treat them with biotoxicity protocols.

Since she'd tested positive for Lyme disease, I prescribed two successive courses of antibiotics to treat the infectious disease. To help reduce the inflammation in her nervous system, I treated her with acupuncture and low-dose naltrexone. She was already eating a clean diet and exercising regularly. Exercise is highly effective in downregulating microglia. So she had been on the right track, but her body had still not been able to sustain itself without collapsing under all the other assaults.

The most alarming result came from the test for inflammation. It showed that Sarah's body had more than six times the normal levels of inflammation. Inflammatory factor C4A should have been at 2,800 or less. Sarah's shot off the chart at 18,000.

Knowing what I know now, I believe the high levels of inflammation in her system were a testament to the accumulation of the physical assaults from the Lyme, biotoxins, and the magnitude of trauma and abuse she had endured at home.

THE ONE-TWO PUNCH OF INFECTION AND TRAUMA

Suspecting that infection and trauma were far more damaging together than either one alone, Urs Meyer, a behavioral neurobiologist in Zurich, and his colleagues ran an unusual study on mice, published in 2013.[18] Infection was easy enough to reproduce, but they couldn't create a specific emotion in mice, so they (quite reasonably) assumed that the stresses of captivity, thirst, and electrocution would be traumatic.

The mothers of one group were dosed with a mild viral infection in late pregnancy. At the age of 6 weeks (early puberty) their offspring were exposed to random stressors: restraining them by force, depriving them of water, and subjecting them to electrical shocks on their feet.[19] In the second group, the mothers were exposed to infection, but the offspring were not subjected to stress. In the third group, the mothers were not exposed to infection, but the offspring were exposed to stress. In the control group, the mothers were not infected, and the offspring were not stressed.

Afterward, the adolescent mice were given a series of behavioral tests to measure the effects. When they reached adulthood (10 weeks), they were tested again. As expected, the mice subjected to early infection combined with stress during puberty had far more behavioral and brain deficits than the others.

Most striking was that the effect was not just cumulative. When infection and stress combined, they acted in synergy. In other words, the impact was greater than the sum of the parts. The anxiety, memory, and cognitive abilities of the mice were far worse.[20]

When the researchers examined the microglia in the brain tissue, the effect was vividly clear. Microglia look like thin, threadlike strands, unless they are upregulated, in which case they swell and change their shape. The microglia in groups exposed to infection or stress alone did not significantly change. In the first group, the activation of the microglia had doubled or tripled in the hippocampus and prefrontal cortex. These are the regions of the brain directly related to depression,[21] posttraumatic stress, and other mood disorders.[22]

Therapists who work with children continually exposed to stress in dysfunctional families often talk about a quality of hypervigilance, a heightened sensitivity to threat. It is one of the criteria for PTSD and is seen in combat veterans, as well as in patients with fibromyalgia and chronic pain.[23]

Meyer's mice showed similar effects. Prepulse inhibition is a neurological test that involves startling the mice with a loud, unexpected noise. Normally, mice and humans are less startled by a noise if there is a warning: a quiet tone a few milliseconds beforehand.

The mice exposed to both infection and stress had become so hypersensitive that even when they were given a warning, they reacted to the loud noise with the same intensity.[24] Raised in the controlled conditions of the lab, these mice had not been stressed since puberty. Yet even as adults, their brains reacted with full alert.

It is just what we would expect from the microglia. Once they have sustained a hyperactivated state, they remember it. They are quicker to flare up and harder to quiet down.

PHYSICAL OUTCOMES, EMOTIONAL PAIN

Chronic physiological hypersensitivity is common in three conditions that often accompany abusive childhoods: irritable bowel syndrome (IBS), post-traumatic stress disorder (PTSD), and depression. The key neurotransmitters may be different, but they each show evidence of sensitization. With IBS, serotonin imbalances are thought to play a role in creating heightened sensitivity to pain. With PTSD, norepinephrine levels are too high. With depression, we see abnormally high levels of cortisol.[25]

Of all pain syndromes, the most obvious connection can be made between abuse and IBS. Anyone with a history of abuse—as a child or an adult—is three times more likely to have IBS.[26] In PTSD, the same hypersensitivity is expressed through flashbacks, acute emotional pain over past traumas, and nightmares. Vulnerability to depression can also be the result of early trauma.[27] An inclination to depression can increase over time, long after the original stimulus has passed.[28]

Psychotherapy can be extremely useful in all cases, since the way a person views a traumatic event can keep it alive, causing that person to relive the original experience. It is almost inevitable for adult survivors of childhood abuse to adopt cognitive distortions about the world.[29] In her classic book, *Trauma and Recovery,* psychiatrist Judith Herman describes the emotional contortions any child in an abusive home has to make:

> Repeated trauma in childhood forms and deforms the personality. The child trapped in an abusive environment is faced with the formidable task of adaptation. She must find a way to preserve a sense of trust in people who are untrustworthy, safety in a situation that is unsafe, control in a situation that is terrifyingly unpredictable, power in a situation of helplessness. Unable to care for or protect herself, she must compensate for the failures of adult care and protection with the only means at her disposal, an immature system of psychological defenses.[30]

As a pain specialist, all of my training and experience confirms that these defenses—which were such an important survival mechanism during the trauma—have to be addressed before a patient can recover full health.

Every patient is different. In general terms, women with a history of sexual abuse often experience more intensive pain, days off work, surgeries, and disability than women who have not been sexually abused. Yet physical abuse of women results in even worse health outcomes.[31]

EFFECTS ON CHILDREN AND ADULTS

While it's long been assumed that the abuse of children has more profound effects than the abuse of adults, the studies show otherwise. Patients who first experience abuse in childhood and those who first experience abuse as adults often experience the same degree of trauma.[32]

Although we have an increasing ability to measure levels of neurotransmitters and other biomarkers, we cannot make easy assumptions about the complicated workings of human emotion, particularly when it comes to dealing with trauma. Ironically, researchers in one study discovered that, when women with a history of physical or sexual assault were raped, they had dramatically lower cortisol responses than women who had never been assaulted.[33] It might seem that they experienced less stress. And yet lower cortisol levels in the face of an assault raised the risk of developing PTSD.[34]

What happened to that stress? Why were their cortisol levels so low? A well-honed ability to detach from all-too-familiar traumas may have been crucial, even lifesaving, in the moment, but it did not appear to offset the consequences of trauma in the long run.

BIOMARKERS FOR MENTAL HEALTH

Evaluating physiological markers is relatively new, but we have come so far that, in 2013, the National Institutes of Mental Health (NIMH) formally stepped away from the subjective measures traditionally used to evaluate psychological disorders. In place of the *Diagnostic and Statistical Manual of Mental Disorders*, the NIMH will create its own diagnostic criteria, based on physiological measurements as opposed to subjective measurements.[35]

With the new, indisputable understanding that mental disorders are biological disorders, they will use genetics, imaging, cognitive science, and other data to create a diagnostic approach based on biology. Because we do not yet know all the biomarkers for psychological issues, the work will be ongoing, but it is a major step in the right direction.

For the most part, psychology has offered subjective, if often well-informed, interpretations. In the hands of a skilled psychotherapist, the diagnosis and its treatment are often priceless. That said, shifting to a physiological lens allows us to think about aberrant emotional states in terms of the activation of microglia. It allows us to ask a whole different set of questions and get a very different set of results.

We have had the taxonomy wrong. Putting mental health issues into boxes has limited our ability to treat people. It was useful for a while and took us to a certain point, but now we can exchange that construct for a more complete model that allows us to treat the whole ecosystem of a person. It was an artificial construct that we had to rely on until we could understand the underlying physiology. It's high time to change that.

When we see psychological conditions in terms of neuroinflammation and neurodegeneration, it changes our whole thought process about what we're looking at and what is the best, most direct way to help them heal.

With this view, the boundaries between psychology and medicine disappear. Suddenly, it becomes obvious why antidepressant drugs work so beautifully for migraines, peripheral neuropathy, or irritable bowel syndrome. It makes sense that antiseizure medications would be effective for peripheral neuropathies, fibromyalgia, and psychiatric diseases. In all of these cases, we are looking at a sensitized, inflamed central nervous system. There is an impairment of common neurophysiological and neuroanatomical pathways. At the cellular level, a hyperreactive nervous system indicates that the microglia have upregulated.

Now we understand how we get sick, why we stay sick, and how we can recover. Because we understand more about how our bodies work, we know how the state of our health has evolved.

AN IMMUNE SYSTEM WEAKENED BY ABUSE

Now we know, for instance, that an immune system weakened in childhood by a pervasive atmosphere of fear, hostility, and abuse in the home is physiologically devastating. Whether that devastation is expressed through pain, depression, disease, mental illness, or a series of unfortunate accidents, it will have a synergistic impact.

People who were traumatized in childhood often bounce back in their twenties, but by the time they reach their thirties and forties, it is as if their bodies have depleted their resilience. Their mental and physical health begins to degrade to a degree that cannot be explained by external assaults or genetics alone. The questions are: How hard has life been? How much resilience is left?

Resilience is nearly impossible to predict. To a large degree, it is entirely individual. Not everyone abused as a child develops chronic pain. There are athletes who suffer repeated injuries and fully recover on their own. We don't often talk about it, but some people who smoke and drink whiskey live well into old age.

Even the scourge of cancer is only contracted in certain ecosystems. Many people do not realize that cancer occurs in our bodies all the time. Cancer cells are often mistakenly made when our bodies reproduce abnormal cells, but our immune system wipes them out. Cell death is a part of the ordinary function of our bodies, as abnormal cells are eliminated. When someone has cancer, it is because the system has malfunctioned and failed to eliminate the abnormal cells. When the immune system is functioning properly, cancer cells are killed as a matter of course.

At 23, Sarah's body is already breaking down. I'm well aware of what can happen to her over the next 10 to 20 years if she does not do this therapy.

It would not be unusual for her to get into the kind of relationships she's most comfortable with. But because she's smart, she'll know to avoid the kind of people who directly resemble her family. Most likely, she'll stay away from people who fly into a rage and throw things. But there are other dysfunctions. She's accustomed to living in an off-balanced environment where she can take up the slack by nurturing others. So, a strong, self-sufficient man could easily make her feel like she has no purpose.

The odds are high that she will live a very stressful life, despite her good intentions. She'll try to eat well and exercise, but her efforts may well be thwarted and she won't really know why. If we're seeing this much breakdown already, it is highly likely that she will experience total incapacity long before she reaches old age.

Physiologically, psychological issues are not separate from pain issues. They are the same thing manifesting differently.

I urged Sarah to consider therapy once again. "I have no interest in you being a doctor," I told her. "I want you to be a healer. So you have to do your own work first."

When she agreed to try therapy, it wasn't easy. She would spend each session in tears and end up with a migraine for the remainder of the day. But now we're talking about true healing. Over time, her microglia will quiet down and she will have a good life and a total recovery.

A PHYSICAL AND EMOTIONAL BREAKTHROUGH

Today Sarah reports that her leg is "98 percent improved." She is no longer in pain every day. Her energy levels have dramatically increased. She is returning to sports and becoming more social again. She is a different person than she was a year ago, when we started.

After enduring several notably unpleasant rounds of IV antibiotics to eliminate the Lyme disease from her system, along with probiotic supplementation, which I always prescribe with antibiotics to protect the gastrointestinal tract, she stopped getting sick every month. In the past year, she had a cold only once. Her fear that her immune system was failing is completely gone.

She recently enrolled in osteopathic medical school. With her interest in medicine, Sarah was particularly astounded by the comprehensive process we went through to get here. "Of all the doctors I've seen, you were the only one who ever took a full medical history of every assault my body has received since I was young. Now I see why!"

It will take some time for her microglia to quiet down. We still have so much to learn, but we do know this: It's not just about stopping the input. It takes a while for the microglia to downregulate. Now that we know their importance, intensive research may reveal new and better ways to manage their regulation.

This is the first big step—a major shift in our thinking, based on the physiology. It is the beginning of a unified theory.

Part III
The Path to Total Recovery

CHAPTER 8

STACKING THE DECK IN YOUR FAVOR

WHAT YOU CAN DO

The only diagnoses you make are those that you make and those that you think of.

Thomas Pinder, MD

The bottom line is: When it comes to chronic pain and depression, there is no reason why you "just have to put up with it." We now know that these states—and a host of conditions that accompany them—are caused by the inflammation of microglia in the brain.

The microglia not only turn on inflammation, but they also remember emotional or physical assaults from the past. We are all at risk. When the microglia in our brains reach a tipping point, they become hyperreactive. The slightest assault can set them off, triggering system-wide inflammation that can be difficult to stop.

I'm encouraged by the brain research currently being done at many of the top medical research centers in the world. My hope is that gaining insight about the connection between microglia upregulation and chronic pain/depression will help speed that work.

As we learn more about the nature of the microglia through the efforts of these scientists, we will find new and better ways to regulate their response to trauma. That information will give us more direct ways to quell the inflammation that results in so many miserable or even fatal conditions.

Depression alone affects 21 million people every year and 51 million over the course of a lifetime.[1] Chronic pain affects more than 100 million.[2] Only recently have we come to realize that so many of our most chronic diseases are primarily inflammatory conditions: inflammatory bowel disease (5 million),[3] cancer (10 million), diabetes (14 million),[4] autoimmune disease (24 million), asthma (30 million), allergies (50 million), rheumatoid arthritis (50 million),[5] and cardiovascular disease (60 million), among many others.

Ideally, we will soon find a way to directly address the underlying mechanism of all these inflammatory diseases. That discovery will revolutionize medicine, dramatically improving and perhaps even eliminating many of these diseases altogether.

In the meantime, we have already developed a powerful, systematic, and highly successful strategy for alleviating chronic pain/depression and its accompanying conditions.

At the Kaplan Center, I've brought together a team that brings a uniquely integrative approach, with specialties in family medicine, pain medicine, physical medicine and rehabilitation, psychological counseling, and medical acupuncture. Unfortunately, in a single book, I can't convey all the insights such a team might have for your specific issues or those of someone you love. What I can do is explain a new way of thinking about pain and make recommendations that will allow you to reduce inflammation, fortify yourself against the inevitable assaults to your health, and get the best professional help you can.

WHAT ARE YOU PUTTING UP WITH NOW?

It still amazes me how many aches and pains patients take for granted. At the most basic level, many people are stiff in the morning when they get out of bed. They're irritable and foggy-headed until they have a second cup of coffee. Since their friends are having the same experience, they joke about "getting older" and assume that what they're feeling is just nature taking its course, that there's nothing they can do about it. But that's not true.

So many of Charlie's college football buddies (Chapter 3) suffered from backaches, joint pain, and other consequences of playing a violent game that he assumed it was normal and something to just put up with. But there was nothing normal about his chronic pain and depression, or his surgeries and constant need for pharmaceutical drugs.

When Emily's orthopedic surgeons (Chapter 2) sent her home from the hospital after her car accident, they made it clear that it was not unusual to experience chronic pain after such a physical trauma and the subsequent reconstructive surgery. Her headaches, depression, and PTSD would not have surprised them either, but those symptoms were clear signs that she had not fully recovered. Why should Emily put up with it?

What are *you* putting up with?

Whatever it is, the research is showing that the time to address it is now, not later. The microglia do not distinguish among different assaults to our health and well-being. Those that go unresolved can lead to a cumulative effect that shows up, one way or another, as chronic pain and depression.

How many assaults have you accumulated already? Are you young and healthy, or struggling with pain and depression? Do you regularly take over-the-counter medications for acid reflux, gas, or constipation? Is there anything you avoid now because of memories of a past trauma that you can't seem to shake? Do you feel anxiety about driving at night? How much do you have to compensate because of chronic pain? Are you pushing yourself to keep going on little sleep, compensating with stimulants, and ignoring the early warnings signs? Or are you already taking action on what you know about how to live a long, healthy life?

EARLY WARNING SIGNS

In the coming months and years, we can anticipate learning more about how to assess the state of the microglia in our brains, but we can already make well-informed deductions. You may be wondering what kind of shape your microglia are in. If they are keeping track of cumulative assaults, how high is the tally? What can you do to improve your odds, to stack the deck in your favor?

If you are healthy now, look for early warning signs in the areas listed below. If you are sick and don't know why, setbacks in these areas may have had a cumulative impact on your health.

In the Resources section on page 213, you'll find a list of tests that will be helpful in assessing your condition. Before I run any tests with my patients, I take a comprehensive history, beginning with questions about the areas that follow. As I gather information about each of these areas, I start to understand their story and make connections that serve as clues to what may have caused and may still be maintaining inflammation in their brain and body.

Quality of Sleep

Sleep is vital to the health of all of our bodily functions in ways that our latest science is making increasingly evident. If you wake up feeling tired in the morning, as if you haven't slept well, it's not something that should be dismissed lightly. Expecting your body to function on too little or poor quality sleep is like expecting it to function without food, water, or oxygen.

It is estimated that approximately 40 million Americans suffer from a chronic sleep disorder.[6] Sleep apnea is one of the most common. It affects more than 5 percent of the population, yet the overwhelming majority of people whose quality of sleep is significantly impaired because of sleep apnea have not been diagnosed.[7]

If you have sleep apnea, you stop breathing episodically throughout the night. Starved for oxygen, your body and brain lapse into a condition known as hypoxia. This means that you spend as much as a third of your day (8 hours out of every 24) in a dangerous, oxygen-deprived state. The ability of your brain, muscles, nerves, and organs to regenerate is diminished. Your body cannot remain in a healthy state if it can't use the time during sleep to repair itself. That's why sleep apnea can take more than 10 years off your life. Literally.

When your blood oxygen levels drop in the night, your body becomes desperate for air. In a state of alarm, your microglia activate. Your adrenals panic, kicking out cortisol—the stress hormone—to wake you up. Maybe you fluff your pillow and go back to sleep. Maybe you go to the bathroom. Either way, you start breathing, which is what your body needs. But when you go back to sleep, the cycle starts all over again. Some people experience it as restlessness. Others find themselves getting up several times at night. None of them is getting the good night's sleep that is so vital to our health and survival.

Considering how hard it is on the body, it's no surprise that sleep apnea causes hypertension, weight gain, type 2 diabetes, and stroke. It is associated with PTSD, anxiety disorders, depression, and chronic pain. It also upregulates microglia, causing inflammation.

People with sleep apnea often snore loudly and never feel rested, even after regularly getting 8 to 9 hours of sleep. Anyone, even children, can suffer from sleep apnea, though men are somewhat more likely than women to develop it. Smoking and being overweight are risk factors, since both can inhibit the ability to breathe well. Anything that obstructs the airway in the throat can create bouts of sleep apnea, from enlarged tonsils to the collapse of the soft tissue walls of the throat during sleep.

Of course, there are a lot of reasons for waking up in the night and even more for feeling tired all day. Complaining about lack of sleep is almost as common as complaining about the weather, but that doesn't mean it's not serious. This is one of those things that everyone dismisses but that can kill you a decade sooner than your family and friends, if you ignore it.

Start by getting at least 7 to 8 hours of sleep a night on a regular basis. Practicing good sleep hygiene will help. Turn off all electronic devices 1 hour before bedtime. Go to bed at about the same time every night and wake up at about the same time, so your body develops a rhythm of rest cycles. Using relaxation or meditation tapes can also be useful.

If you still sleep poorly—snoring, getting up in the night, tossing and turning, or waking up feeling tired—recognize that it is an unnecessary health problem that needs to be addressed. If you suspect you have sleep apnea, the simplest diagnosis is the home WatchPAT test (see Resources), which I use with my patients. There are several other home tests available through your doctor. If you have any reason to believe that you might have sleep issues, get tested as soon as possible. If there is a problem, you could be losing hours of sleep every night. You'll be amazed by how much better it feels to wake up truly rested.

Infections and Antibiotics

All infections, by definition, create an inflammatory state in the body, but not all of them trigger microglial inflammation. Bacteria on the skin will incite a reaction to kill it, remove it, and regenerate tissue. This process is mediated by white cells, not the microglia. Allergies provoke an inflammatory reaction and the release of histamines, which cause itchy eyes, runny nose, and asthma. Allergies can, but don't necessarily, activate the microglia.

Any time pain, fever, malaise, mood alterations, and general inflammation occur together, it's a sign that the central nervous system is engaged. That tells us that the microglia have gotten involved.

As I have said, the body is an ecosystem, so inflammation in the periphery can always potentially affect the central nervous system as well. The extent to which that inflammation crosses over depends on the health of the individual and the level of reactivity of the microglia in their brain.

A lingering infection in the body can perpetuate inflammation—gingivitis, Lyme disease, and other tick-borne illnesses are a few examples of infections that can have such an impact. Complete eradication of these conditions can make a significant difference.

Ironically, the treatments we use often cause more inflammation than the infections themselves. Doctors often prescribe antibiotics for infections of the sinuses, bronchial tubes, and teeth. Multiple treatments of antibiotics for any reason can profoundly change the gut flora. Those changes can then damage the intestinal tract enough to create leaky gut syndrome, which will result in inflammation and activate the microglia. Taking live probiotics can help replenish the flora. While a recommendation of probiotics is not yet the standard of practice in medicine, there is increasing evidence that it should be. The good news is probiotics are available without a medical prescription. I'll talk more about probiotics in the section on supplements (see page 198).

It's not that antibiotics are bad. Before we had antibiotics, some infections that are relatively minor today escalated into life-threatening illnesses. But we also know that antibiotics can have damaging side effects, especially on the balance of intestinal bacteria, so it makes sense to be aware of the consequences of using them—particularly of taking them frequently—and take precautions to offset it.

Physical Trauma

Most people recover readily from broken bones, concussions, sprained ankles, and other physical traumas. Our bodies are designed to repair themselves in remarkable ways. At this stage of our knowledge about the microglia, it seems that as long as we fully recover from physical traumas, they do not become part of the cumulative buildup that can provoke relentless inflammation.

The injuries that contribute to that assault overload seem to be the ones that have never fully healed. When patients tell me they had an injury, particularly a minor one, and it's been "a problem ever since," I start thinking about microglia.

Chronic pain is one of the clearest signs of upregulated microglia, whether the pain is low-grade or severe. With every patient in this book—and dozens that I see in my offices every week—an ongoing state of upregulated microglia resulted in serious illnesses that were much harder to treat at that later stage. If they had been nipped in the bud earlier, the patients would have suffered far less.

All of us are in the habit of dismissing our minor aches and pains. Over time, we learn ways to work around a "trick knee" or "bad back." If the pain is not enough to interfere with our sleep or our daily lives, we tend to put up with it, especially if our doctor tells us it's something we'll "just have to live with."

We find ways to ease the pain—a special pillow, ice packs, massagers, or heating pads. No one thinks twice about popping an NSAID, so we easily get in the habit of taking them, not realizing how much they may be impairing our health. Remember, NSAIDs damage the cells lining the intestines in the majority of people who take them. They are anti-inflammatory, but they do nothing to affect the underlying disease. Taking them once in a while is probably not a problem, because the gut can heal, but with consistent long-term use, you could be creating a serious imbalance of gut flora.

If you still feel lingering effects from a physical trauma, I encourage you to find a way to treat it. Total recovery is your best protection against the effects of cumulative traumas. Bone, joint, and muscle issues can often be successfully treated with physical therapy, acupuncture, musculoskeletal manipulation, and/or prolotherapy.

Psychological Trauma

Lingering psychological traumas are every bit as damaging as physical traumas. Whether or not you cry is not a good measure of the impact of an emotionally charged situation. People living in chronically abusive situations quickly learn to suppress their feelings in an effort to cope. Traumatic emotional experiences can live in the body with every bit as much virulence and danger as an untreated wound.

A soldier in battle, a child with a pathological parent, a spouse of an alcoholic, an accident survivor, or a victim of a tsunami all experience trauma but deal with it in radically different ways. Again, the sign that should concern you is any trauma that lingers, whether you believe it ought to linger or not.

We've all had emotional traumas. It's part of life. If you wonder about your own, look for clues that tell you you're not over it. Where has your fear of something made you rigid? Which painful memories make you overreact?

If you have truly recovered from a painful trauma from the past, you will find you're more resilient when you experience a similar trauma again. It was more upsetting the first time, but now you're stronger. It was shocking then, but now you're not surprised at all. Even dramatic upheavals are more manageable now, if you have genuinely come to terms with whatever happened before.

That is what emotional recovery looks like. Lack of recovery is very different. Because unhealed trauma is like an untreated wound, it leaves you far more vulnerable to future assaults. Instead of improving your resilience, it undermines your physical and emotional health. As it lingers in the body, it sustains the upregulation of the microglia, leaving you open to the buildup of cumulative assaults you're hoping to avoid. It may show up as avoidance or emotional overreaction to certain situations, and may even reach the level of post-traumatic stress disorder, anxiety disorder, or major depression.

Depending on the nature of the trauma and your willingness to move past it, you may find a variety of solutions helpful. At the simplest level, confiding in friends can often provide the balm that's needed for emotional pain. A carefully selected therapist or psychiatrist can provide longer-term, more empirically considered options. To some degree, practices that shift the energy in the body can reduce the impact of a physical trauma. Meditation, massage, acupuncture, and many forms of exercise can all help.

Keep in mind that lingering issues literally put your health at risk. Now that we know these issues can be cumulative, do whatever you can to alleviate that pain.

Nutritional and Gastrointestinal Issues

Obesity, celiac disease, gluten intolerance, allergies, and leaky gut fall into this category. I always ask my patients to answer these questions:

- How is your digestion?
- Do you have any food sensitivities?
- Have you experienced brain fog after eating certain foods?
- Do you have bloating or gas?
- Do you experience regular or episodic constipation or diarrhea?
- Do you have acid reflux?
- Do you have problems with abdominal pain?
- Are you taking a proton pump inhibitor or digestive aid?
- Have you had episodes of gastroenteritis?
- Have you developed severe diarrhea while traveling?
- Have you ever been significantly overweight?

Patients who are obese or overweight have an inflammatory condition that predisposes them not only to type 2 diabetes and heart disease, but also to chronic pain and depression. More than 65 percent of Americans are overweight.[8] This is a health risk factor we must control.

Gas, bloating, and poor digestion are also so common in our culture that it's easy to assume they're normal and nothing to worry about. Regular gastrointestinal discomfort—even minor discomfort—is not normal. It may be a symptom of a sustained inflammatory reaction in your body due to leaky gut, celiac disease, gluten intolerance, or other gastrointestinal disorders. (If you see fat droplets or blood in your stool, it requires a prompt evaluation.)

If you experience regular indigestion, start with the dietary recommendations later in this chapter. If these simple interventions don't resolve the problem, find a doctor who will do a proper medical workup to evaluate your concerns.

Medications

Because of the powerful, short-term effectiveness of many drugs, we're beginning to experience polypharmaceutical problems, where patients end up taking one drug to treat the side effects of other drugs.

With the rise of specialization, doctors are not always aware of which drugs their patients are taking, much less their side effects. I've seen doctors give proton pump inhibitors (for gastric issues) to patients with orthopedic problems, not realizing that those drugs increase the risk of fractures.

Stomach acid is necessary for normal digestion of food. It is our first line of defense against bacteria and viruses that may be ingested with our food. Medications that reduce stomach acid have been associated with magnesium and B_{12} deficiencies, bacterial overgrowth of the intestines, and an increased risk of developing pneumonia.[9] Here are only a few examples of the ramifications of common medications.

- **Statins.** This common group of medications is used to treat elevated cholesterol. They can be the cause of cataracts and unexplained muscle pain.[10, 11] Some studies show they may increase your risk of developing diabetes.[12]
- **NSAIDs.** Frequent use of NSAIDs can increase gastritis, acid

reflux, gas, and bloating. More than 70 percent of people chronically taking NSAIDs—such as ibuprofen (Advil, Motrin), naproxen (Naprosyn), diclofenac (Voltaren), and aspirin (Bayer, Bufferin)—will get ulcers in their small intestines, creating a permeability problem (aka leaky gut syndrome).[13]

- **Opioids.** These painkillers—such as codeine, hydrocodone (Vicodin), morphine (Avinza), and oxycodone (Percocet)—can lead to depression, constipation, and sexual dysfunction and actually heighten sensitivity to pain.[14]
- **Sleeping pills.** A chronic reliance on any type of sleeping pill—such as zolpidem (Ambien), eszopiclone (Lunesta), or zaleplon (Sonata)—can, in the short term, make it hard to focus and, in the long run, even shorten your life span. Among the elderly, sleeping pills can increase the risk of falls and fractures.[15]

The rough guideline I give my patients about taking medications is this: A drug has to work better than the side effects it creates. If it doesn't, get rid of it.

Naturally, you may need to do so under the supervision of a doctor. It often takes months, even up to a year, to wean patients off of strong medications. Benzodiazepines—such as diazepam (Valium), alprazolam (Xanax), clonazepam (Klonopin), and lorazepam (Ativan)—can cause anxiety, panic attacks, hallucinations, seizures, and psychoses for months or even years after a patient stops taking them, if they are not reduced slowly enough.[16]

The truth is, we can frequently find better—more effective, less toxic—solutions with few, if any, side effects to take their place. Often, I find that people are taking medications simply because they were prescribed, whether they are working or not. Know why you are taking medications and make sure they are working for you. If you decide to look for alternatives, don't just stop a prescription medication. Check with your doctor.

By addressing the early warning signs, we are attempting to remove everything that can potentially put the microglia in a chronic inflammatory state, even though the causes of inflammation are gone. Making a timeline of your history, which I'll explain below, can help you and your doctor identify the assaults and traumas your body has already endured that may be affecting your health today.

WHAT IS STACKING THE DECK AGAINST YOU?

If you already have a pretty healthy lifestyle, you have been stacking the deck in your favor. At the same time, of course, none of us comes through life unscathed. We have all survived a series of major and minor traumas. Sometimes they have made us stronger, but that is not always the case.

As a physician, I believe it is my job to help identify the clues to my patients' conditions. No matter what their initial symptoms are, I start by asking, "When was the last time you felt completely healthy, vital, and strong?"

The first thing most people do is lie to me.

"I was in excellent health until that car accident 5 years ago."

"I felt strong and healthy until my sophomore year, when that headache came over me in the middle of class."

"I was always healthy until after the birth of my second child."

They tell me about a traumatic or infectious event, not realizing that their current condition is far more complex. Their symptoms may have started with an event, but most are the result of a process. A cumulative series of events gradually undermined their health until their body couldn't recover from the "event" that they think caused the problem. So, unwittingly, they lie.

We start where they want to start, but as their stories unfold, it inevitably turns out that they have had a long history of aches and pains. But they assumed that was normal. As seemingly minor problems became chronic, they figured they'd "just have to live with them." After all, a lot of their friends complained of the same sort of thing.

"Your back pain started after you moved that furniture around, but how is your sleep?" I ask a patient.

"Oh, I really haven't slept well since I was a child," she shrugs.

"Fatigue is your main concern," I say, acknowledging another patient's complaint. "But do you ever get headaches?"

"I've had migraines two to three times a month since I was a teenager, but I take medication and they go away," he tells me.

What I see as a problem is very different from what my patients see. As you've read in this book, I bring a very different perspective. I know only too well that the physical and emotional traumas we endure are cumulative. Everything's related. And we have to know what's happened and evaluate whether it's relevant, so we can follow the trail.

Having a doctor evaluate those connections is ideal, but you can start with a timeline and begin to make notes about the kind of connections you've learned about from reading this book. A doctor who knows what to make of your story can glean invaluable insight from your timeline. If your own doctor does not approach medicine this way, you can find doctors that do (see Resources, page 211).

Your Timeline

The goal is to develop a timeline of life events and health issues to see if a cumulative pattern emerges or to find evidence of how an illness evolved over the years. Inevitably, it is an ongoing process, as the patient remembers things, and we explore the connections together.

Our results are so persuasive that my patients' perspectives begin to change simply by seeing their health histories before their eyes. Before long, they learn to notice connections themselves.

You can do the same by developing your own timeline to track the chronology. Create three columns titled Major Life Events, Emotional Traumas and Stresses, and Physical Traumas and Issues. You can fill in positive changes and happy events in your life in a fourth column, as well.

On my Web site—www.kaplanclinic.com—I have provided timeline software that will make it easy for you to fill in the events and make connections between them. You can also use tables on your computer, create transparencies to overlay the categories, or write out the timeline on a big sheet of paper. The important thing is to write down as much as you can remember and start to notice what changed for you after each major event.

Major Life Events

Starting with the day you were born, list the significant events in your life by year in chronological order. Include different places you have lived, births (yourself, your siblings, and your own children), marriages, divorces (your parents' or your own), graduations, jobs, military service, travel history, and deaths of loved ones. Joyous events, like a marriage, the birth of a child, or a move to a wonderful new home, can be stressful, just like traumas are. All of the significant events should be listed.

In 1967, the Holmes-Rahe Stress Inventory was created by two psychiatrists, Thomas Holmes and Richard Rahe. They correlated the medical records of 5,000 patients, then asked the patients to say how stressful they found each one of 43 stressful life events—such as the death of a spouse, a major personal injury or illness, retirement, major change in the health of a family member, pregnancy, sexual difficulties, taking on a mortgage, a child leaving home, an outstanding personal achievement, changes in residence, changes in eating habits, etc.[17] It may be helpful to start with this inventory, as you recall events from your own life. You can find it at www.stress.org/holmes-rahe-stress-inventory.

Emotional Traumas and Stresses

Has depression or anxiety been an issue for you? Were there significant losses in your life or times when you were under extraordinary stress?

It is important to note the dates of significant emotional stressors—when they started and whether they are ongoing. If you grew up in an emotionally or physically abusive household, or were involved in an abusive relationship, it goes in this column. If you have had a history of drug or alcohol abuse issues, this is the place to list them. Prolonged stressful periods due to finances, illnesses, sexual issues, family pressures, relationships, or outside influences of any kind can cause significant emotional reactions in the body.

Everyone reacts differently to traumas and stresses. You may have experienced all of these things, but fully recovered. What's most important is to focus on anything that lingers. What are you having trouble letting go of?

Physical Traumas and Issues

List in chronological order the onset and dates of all significant illnesses. Include ongoing and intermittent problems, such as headaches, sleep issues, aches and pains, or digestive issues. Have you had recurrent infections that required multiple courses of antibiotics? If so, list the dates and duration.

Do not forget to include any and all of the early warning signs.

Any significant accidents, physical traumas, surgeries, or hospitalizations go in this column. If you have taken medications, describe when you started them, why, when you stopped, and any significant side effects.

Include any exposure to environmental toxins you may have had, too. In the places where you have lived, was there any water or mold damage? Were you regularly exposed to cigarette smoke, or did you smoke? Write down the dates and amounts.

When you have completed all three columns, step back and look them over. The connections may surprise you. If the microglia are involved, there will be a relationship between inflammatory events.

Now that you have the timeline before you, your detective work can begin. Your goal is to make the connections that reveal the story of your health. Remember that all of these events have had an impact on the ecosystem of your body. Look for the clues that tell you which ones were resolved and which ones laid the groundwork for things to come.

Ask yourself how life started out for you. Was your home environment safe? When did the trouble start? How old were you? What happened next? How was your sleep? Did you have pain, depression, anxiety, intestinal disorders? When did you first notice any problems with energy, focus, or concentration? What incidents signaled a decline in your health: a pregnancy, accident, injury, loss, or emotional blow?

You may have never associated these events with the overall state of your health before, but that's okay. You are learning to see the connections, to recognize what they cost in the long run and how they can leave you vulnerable if they are not resolved.

Your health is an evolutionary process with symptoms and events emerging from one another. You can improve it or impair it as you go.

Making connections with the timeline allows you to see your symptoms in the context of your life. Those connections are the key to how you got sick, why you stay sick, and how you can recover.

Positive Changes and Happy Events

While you're making your timelines of traumas and health issues, keep track of the healthy behavioral changes and new habits you've developed, too. You can even make a new column for the positive developments and track their influence on your health and well-being. It is encouraging to see positive patterns emerge. Your actions have the ability to build deep strength and resilience into your body for the long term. They generate a cumulative sense of health and well-being that is not always dramatic, but moves you steadily in the right direction.

By being attentive, you can notice the positive changes. Did your energy increase 6 weeks after you gave up smoking? Has eating more fresh vegetables improved your immune system so much that you haven't caught a cold in 2 years? Everything you do to reduce inflammation and fortify your health actively gives you an advantage.

HOW TO STACK THE DECK IN YOUR FAVOR

With our new understanding of microglia, we have more reason than ever to eat well, exercise, meditate, and make sure our bodies have the nutrients they need. There is no way for us to entirely avoid the stresses and traumas life brings, but we can take action that will enable us to recover more quickly when they occur and intercede when the effects become chronic.

Try a Low-Inflammatory Diet

One of the first things I recommend to all of my patients with microglial inflammation is a plan to eliminate any foods from their diets that are likely culprits for allergies or sensitivities.

For 6 weeks, they eat only brown rice, fish, chicken, eggs, fresh fruits, and vegetables. This diet eliminates the most frequent foods people are allergic or sensitive to, such as wheat, soy, milk, and milk products. The hormones and antibiotics in commercial beef are a problem, but truly organic, grass-fed beef can be included in the diet.

Breakfast tends to be the most challenging meal on this diet. In addition to eggs, include fresh fruits and vegetables with this meal. Smoothies with protein powder (not soy based) are a good choice, as are fish such as salmon or herring.

If you have food sensitivities, omit the foods you know about. This diet will not eliminate every food that you're sensitive to. That will be a process of discovery as you go along. If you have been living with sluggishness and brain fog, the diet will help to remove a large number of foods that may have been causing those symptoms.

After following this diet for a few weeks, my patients often identify allergies and sensitivities to foods they never suspected were creating problems. These issues quickly become conspicuous. And when those foods that were causing their bodies to respond with inflammation are removed, they are surprised by the increase in energy and mental clarity.

Start an "Eating and Aftereffects" Diary

On this diet, it is important to keep a food diary. In addition to writing down what you eat and when you eat it, you will also check back in with yourself in intervals throughout the day to see how the food made you feel. For example, did you notice nasal congestion, brain fog, sluggishness, bloating, or a headache after eating certain foods?

Allergies and food sensitivities may not show up for hours after you eat the offending food or spice. But if you are alert, your odds of making connections between the food and your response improve. With such a clean diet, it is easy to notice if you have a harder time concentrating after you eat a certain food. Getting in the habit of paying attention to the effects food have on you is also a valuable skill for the future.

Be sure to write down exactly how you feel at the beginning of the diet, so you can make an accurate comparison in 6 weeks.

Avoid Stimulants

No one is happy when I say that they will have to give up all stimulants for 6 weeks. That means no caffeinated coffee, tea, or alcohol. It means no NSAIDs to inflame your gut. If you typically drink more than two cups of coffee a day, your body may be addicted and you might get a withdrawal headache when you give it up. I recommend cutting your consumption in half every few days. If you normally drink six cups of coffee, cut it down to three cups (or six cups of half-caff). A few days later, cut it down to 1.5 cups for a few days. After a week or two of easing off caffeine, you should be able to go without coffee and not get a headache.

Evaluate Your Progress

Recording your health in your food diary is an important component of this diet. But let's keep it simple. Before you start the diet, and weekly thereafter, rate the following factors in your diary. You can use a single number or a general range:

- Your energy level: 1–10 (10 is ideal)
- Your ability to focus and concentrate: 1–10 (10 is ideal)
- Your general pain level: 1–10 (10 is severe pain)
- Your specific pain level for chronic incidents, such as headaches or migraines, and how many days you experience them: 1–10 (10 is severe)

It is best to complete the diary at the same time every day. As a rule, I have my patients complete the diary at the end of their day. Feel free to add comments about your sleep, digestion, or any other aspect of your health and mood. Make note of any unusual major life events.

Do not review the weekly diary until you have completed all 6 weeks of the diet. Looking at last week's entry may influence what you write this week. It's best to write down how you are feeling about the most recent week independently of the other weeks.

Add Other Foods One at a Time

After 6 weeks, gradually add other categories of food, one at a time, one week at a time. Many of my patients add dairy back in for the first week, paying close attention to whether it causes gas, bloating, or other reactions. The following week, they may reintroduce soy products, such as tofu, soybeans, miso, and soy sauce. The next week, add wheat, such as bread, cereal, pasta, and canned or frozen foods with wheat fillers. You are the best judge of whether these foods have a negative effect on your energy levels, your mood, or your ability to concentrate.

Look for Signs of Allergies

If you lose as much as 5 pounds or more the first week, it may be a sign that you've been eating foods you're allergic to and your tissues have been swollen. Remember, we are not restricting calories on this diet, just the sources of those calories. My patients frequently do lose weight following it, but if they are not overweight and have not been eating excessive calories, then weight loss for the whole 6 weeks is usually only 3 to 5 pounds.

Other signs of allergies include migraines, numbness in the arms or legs, inability to focus, poor concentration, fatigue, depression, brain fog, headaches, mood fluctuations, itchiness, sneezing, gas, diarrhea, sinus congestion, and skin rashes. Watch for these symptoms. Sometimes they're so familiar they're easy to dismiss, but all of them can indicate an allergic response.

Delayed reactions are not uncommon. You may get a headache in the morning from something you ate last night or find it hard to concentrate hours after being exposed to an allergen. This is one of the reasons for adding foods back into your diet very slowly.

Prepare for the Toughest Part

My patients tell me that the first 2 weeks are the hardest. Old habits can be tough to change. The next most difficult part comes at the end, after the 6 weeks, when they are feeling better but start adding things back in. It's a sad moment when they realize that they're having a reaction to one of their favorite foods. Maybe they add in gluten for few days but soon experience the bloating, congestion, and brain fog they used to think was normal. The signs are obvious, yet almost everyone asks: "Does this mean I can't eat wheat anymore?!"

I tell them what I'll tell you. You can eat whatever you want. It depends on whether you're willing to accept the consequences. But it's up to you.

Consider Supplementation

It is estimated that 92 percent of Americans may have deficiencies of essential vitamins and minerals. Nearly 80 percent are deficient in vitamin D. Almost everyone (99 percent) is deficient in omega-3 fatty acids.[18] Although there is controversy about taking multivitamins, they can be a reliable means of supplementing nutrients missing from the diet.

To counteract microglial inflammation, pay particular attention to magnesium, vitamin D, and omega-3 oils for their anti-inflammatory effects.

Magnesium

Sixty-eight percent of American adults consume less than the Recommended Dietary Allowance (RDA) of magnesium (310–400 milligrams daily), and 19 percent consume less than half of the RDA.[19] Foods with high magnesium content include spinach (1 cup, 160 milligrams), black beans (1 cup, 120 milligrams), edamame (1 cup, 100 milligrams), and almonds (1 ounce, 80 milligrams). But only 30 to 40 percent of dietary magnesium is absorbed by the body.[20]

Magnesium is essential for numerous bodily functions, but it is especially important for controlling the activity of glutamate and excitatory neurotransmitter. People with a magnesium deficiency are more likely to have chronic pain as a result of failure to regulate glutamate activity.

As I discussed earlier, there is specific testing available to measure whole body stores of magnesium. For my patients in whom we have identified a significant magnesium deficiency, we frequently will recommend intravenous replacement. Magnesium can also be taken orally at home. Because it has an irritating effect on the gut and may cause diarrhea, it is best to start with a smaller dose and work up to 150 to 350 milligrams a day of magnesium citrate or glycinate.

Vitamin D

Vitamin D deficiency is a pandemic. Very few foods in our diet provide enough vitamin D. Breads, cereals, and other products fortified with vitamin D are often inadequate. Sun exposure is the main way we synthesize this vitamin.[21]

Since as many as 80 percent of adults have deficient blood levels of vitamin D, supplementation is advisable. It is important to take a biologically active form of the vitamin, known as vitamin D_3 (cholecalciferol). Many vitamin D supplements use vitamin D_2, which is not active.[22] In general, a daily dose of vitamin D_3 2000 IU is sufficient.

To determine the precise dose, you would ask your doctor to monitor your vitamin D status as part of your regular checkup. The ideal blood range is 50 to 80 nanograms per milliliter. If your levels are lower, you may be advised to take a higher dose for a limited period of time, under your doctor's supervision. It can take 6 to 10 months to compensate for a deficiency.[23]

Omega-3s

Omega-3 fatty acids are essential to our health, especially our heart and brain, yet they are not made in the body. We have to get them from our diets. EPA and DHA are derived primarily from fish and packaged in fish oil capsules, while ALA comes from plants and is then converted into EPA and DHA. (DHA can also be found in blue-green algae, though there have been recent reports that it may damage the central nervous system.)[24]

It can be a challenge to find a pure, high-quality fish oil because of the risk of contamination. Dr. Barry Sears, author of *The Omega Rx Zone*, points out that we have dumped mercury, dioxins, and PCBs into the ocean for two generations and have by now contaminated every fish on earth.[25] As a result, the vast majority of fish oil supplements are suspect.[26]

Five years ago, new manufacturing techniques were developed that led to ultrarefined, pharmaceutical-grade EPA/DHA concentrates. The International Fish Oil Standards (IFOS) Program tests the levels of toxins in fish oil samples provided by manufacturers and lists them on its Web site, www.ifosprogram.com/consumer-reports.aspx. Before you choose an omega oil supplement, be sure to confirm that it is free from toxins.[27]

Another way to test the oil is to place the liquid in the freezer. (Cut the capsules open and freeze the oil.) If it freezes solid, it is not the highly refined oil that is likely to be toxin free.[28] If it stays liquid or mushy, it does not mean it's free from contaminants, but it's better than the alternative.

Dr. Sears is renowned for his recommendations of daily high-dose omega-3 oils to combat inflammation:

No chronic disease	2.5 g
Obesity, heart disease, type 2 diabetes	5 g
Chronic pain	7.5 g
Neurological conditions	10 g or more[29]

The body is a complex ecosystem. No one supplement or pill can cure inflammation or prevent the microglia from upregulating. Instead, it's about doing everything you can to stack the deck in your favor.

Probiotics

Throughout the book, I've talked about prescribing live probiotics to help restore the health of the gut, aid in the digestion and assimilation of food, and maintain a proper balance of bacteria in the digestive tract.

The typical American diet doesn't include a lot of food that contains probiotics, such as sauerkraut and Korean kimchi. I recommend that all of my patients on antibiotics take a probiotic while they are on it and for several weeks after they have completed their course of antibiotics, to protect the gut.

If you find the probiotics on the shelf of the health food store, unrefrigerated, most likely they are not alive. While there is some benefit from the DNA of probiotics that are not alive, studies indicate that taking live probiotics confers far better benefits in the improvement of gut health. I take them every day myself and encourage my patients to do the same.

To restore the gut, you will need at least 10,000 to 25,000 CFUs (colony forming units). Pay attention to how it makes you feel. If it gives you diarrhea, reduce the dose. Do you see a reduction of gas, constipation, and bloating? Bowel movements should be rebalanced.

Dark Chocolate

Dark chocolate with 70 percent cocoa contains flavonols with antioxidant and anti-inflammatory properties. In moderate doses (1.5 ounces), it can improve your mood, as well as your LDL and HDL cholesterol levels.[30]

Green Tea

Green tea has been shown to lower LDLs (low-density lipoproteins), which are associated with inflammation in the heart. A 5-year study by the American Heart Association found that when patients with a history of heart attacks drank more than two cups of green tea a day, they lowered their risk of death from a heart attack by 44 percent.[31] A cup of green tea contains more flavonoids than the same amount of fresh fruits, vegetables, or wine.[32]

Exercise Regularly

Most likely, you've known for as long as you can remember that exercise is good for you. Did you know that it also downregulates microglia in the brain?[33]

Exercise not only gives you more energy, but it also reduces brain inflammation—provided you don't overdo it. While you exercise, you need to keep your pulse within 50 to 85 percent of your maximum heart rate rather than strive for a higher intensity.

As Tom Venuto, fitness trainer and bestselling author, points out, "Intensity is relative. If you're a sedentary beginner, walking up one flight of stairs can leave you gasping for air with your heart pounding, so that would be intense, relatively speaking. If you're highly conditioned, a 10-K run could be a breeze."[34]

The traditional way to determine your maximum heart rate (MHR) in beats per minute uses this formula: 220 − your age. If you are sedentary and just starting an exercise regimen, keep your heart rate between 50 and 65 percent of your MHR (220 − your age × 0.50 to 0.65). If you exercise regularly, aim for 60 to 75 percent of your MHR. If you are very active, go for 70 to 85 percent. (If you are taking beta blockers, it will be hard to raise your heart rate. In that case, talk to your doctor about being able to exercise until you build up a light sweat.)

Heart rate monitors are available to tell you exactly how fast your heart is beating. You can also take your own pulse for 10 seconds and multiply it by 6.

Meditate Daily

Meditation has long been used in certain traditions to focus the mind and calm the body. Until recently, however, there was no real biomedical evidence that it could improve health.

Now studies have shown that meditation has a significant and measurable impact on heart disease, back pain, headaches, insomnia, hypertension, arthritis, and many other conditions.[35] Inflammation and emotional reactivity can also be reduced.[36] Meditation has even been proved to increase bloodflow to the brain.[37] Over time, those who practice emotion-oriented meditation, such as loving-kindness meditation, actually increase the gray matter volume in their brains in areas related to emotion.[38]

The evidence in dozens of journals is so substantial that there can be no doubt of meditation's benefits: Meditation is neuroregenerative. The regular practice of any type of meditation will help lower inflammation. Many of my patients are surprised by what a difference it makes. I do it every day myself.

If you're genuinely committed to improving your health, I recommend that you try it. If you meditate 20 minutes a day (or 10 minutes twice a day) for 8 weeks, you may substantially decrease your pain, while improving your mood, your sleep, and your quality of life.

There are many types of meditation. On my Web site (www.kaplanclinic.com) you will find references for several excellent books on the subject. You can also download meditation exercises. Choose any one that feels right to you.

If you prefer, you can adopt a simple breathing exercise instead, allowing your body to gradually relax as you focus on your breath, slowly inhaling, then exhaling, for 20 minutes a day. Thanks to medical research, we know meditation is far more than a calming exercise; it actually reduces inflammation and improves our health.

Inquire about These Promising Medications

When there is pain in a joint, NSAIDs can help reduce the inflammation, but microglial inflammation is different. So far, only a few medications have shown promise.

- **Low-dose naltrexone**[39] (an opioid antagonist, 4.5 milligrams)
- **Minocycline**[40] (a broad spectrum antibiotic)
- **Angiotensin II receptor blocker**[41] (lowers blood pressure)

All three have been shown to keep the microglia from producing inflammatory products in the body. Once we're able to do further research on drugs that can specifically reduce the upregulation of microglia, we will have better choices.

At this early stage, the ideal circumstances under which each of these drugs might be most useful in reducing neuroinflammation is unclear. There is a suggestion that minocycline might do the most in limiting the damage after a stroke. Low-dose naltrexone has proved most beneficial in people with symptoms of chronic fatigue and fibromyalgia. At this time, the research on angiotensin receptor blockers is limited to animal studies and is too new to inform us as to how they might best be used for microglial regulation in humans.

Because of the complexity of microglial physiology, there are a wide range of medications that could potentially have an impact— just as there are a wide range of conditions that result from the chronic upregulation of microglia. As our understanding grows, we will be able to get a much clearer idea about the medications that will help most, even in off-label applications.

Research shows that these three have potential, but the beauty is, now that we know where to look, we may be able to find a lot of medications to address this problem. In the meantime, the only one I prescribe regularly for my patients is low-dose naltrexone.

Let your doctor evaluate the application of these. If necessary, print out the new studies for these drugs that I've included in the endnotes and take them to your appointment. These are recent developments. You cannot expect any doctor to know about everything, but you do need a doctor who will partner with you. At the Kaplan Center, our patients educate us all the time, bringing us new information. We evaluate it. We don't do all of it, but we listen.

TAKE CHARGE OF YOUR HEALTH

The good news is, you can take charge of your own health and start making a difference today. Give priority to your diet. Get your heart rate up for at least 30 minutes a day, every day. Be attentive to your sleep. If you are not waking rested, find out why. Meditate 20 minutes a day or at least do some deep breathing in a quiet space.

When you evaluate your timeline, raise questions. Make notes to yourself about things that should be addressed. Why live in pain and poor health—now or 20 years from now—because of cumulative assaults that could have been fully resolved?

You cannot do it all alone. You will need a partner. Begin a conversation with your health care provider about how you can achieve a total recovery. If your current physician won't partner with you, contact the organizations under "Finding a Doctor" in Resources and ask for their recommendations for doctors in your area. Keep looking until you find one who can help. If you wonder whether you have gluten intolerance, Lyme disease, or some of the other issues mentioned in this book, look over the tests I recommend in "Getting the Right Tests" on page 213, then discuss them with your doctor.

Whether you are suffering from pain and depression, or whether you feel good but want to stay as healthy as possible, you can start stacking the deck in your favor today.

CONCLUSION

A GAME-CHANGING INSIGHT

WHAT IT ALL MEANS

Working scientists . . . don't stop at the facts; they begin there, right beyond the facts, where the facts run out.

Stuart Firestein

In the last 5 years, we have understood more about the workings of disease—the actual physiology—than we have in the previous 20 years. Even now, we are on the brink of major breakthroughs in our fundamental understanding of how the body works in at least five or six medical fields.

The discovery of the microglia connections has given us a way to unite the insights of osteopathic medicine, family medicine, pain management, ancient Chinese medicine, psychology, trigger point therapy, prolotherapy, and a host of alternative and complementary medicines.

Suddenly, everything fits. When microglia upregulate, they create widespread inflammation in the brain. If they are turned on too often, they become hyperreactive.

Considering the body's limited range of expression, their reaction isn't nuanced. Like a toggle switch, the microglia turn on or off. Every injury, every infection, every toxin, every trauma, every emotional blow generates the same reaction. Inside the brain, it triggers the microglia again and again and again. The more frequently the microglia are triggered, the more sensitive they become to the next stimulus. Finally, there comes a point when the microglia remain in an upregulated state, causing neuroinflammation long after the stimulus is gone.

What this means is that the traumas we suffer have a cumulative effect. Instead of looking at the outcome—neurological diseases, autoimmune disorders, psychological problems, chronic illnesses of all kinds—it is imperative that we learn to recognize the clues leading up to them.

When we understand that disease is not an event but a process, it makes sense that a 30-year-old woman who is raped as a child and gets a concussion from a car accident in her twenties could develop debilitating fibromyalgia and clinical depression. These events may seem unrelated, but all of them upregulate microglia, resulting in a chronic neuroinflammatory condition.

When an economics major in college, who has finally escaped the clutches of his violent alcoholic father, strains his back while moving into the dorm and the pain keeps coming back at the slightest provocation, it's understandable. With constant emotional abuse, the inflammatory factors in his brain have become hyperreactive. Even a minor injury can lead to chronic pain if the inflammation never subsides. The chronic pain he feels is not from the injury; it's from the chronic inflammatory state created by years of emotional abuse. The injury is only the tipping point.

Knowing how microglia work allows us to connect the dots. Now we can see disease for what it is: the outcome of our life experiences.

Until now, our best options were to mask the symptoms. For the first time in history, we are on the threshold of knowing how to cure them. By quelling inflammation at its source—inside the brain—we can finally have success with such diverse and chronic conditions, such as fibromyalgia, migraines, osteoarthritis, back pain, neuropathy, depression, post-traumatic stress disorder, anxiety disorders, irritable bowel syndrome, and many more.

In recent years, dozens of popular books have been published on autoimmune disease and anti-inflammatory diets for everything from hay fever to autism, as the public has become more aware of the dangers of inflammation. Knowing what we know about leaky gut and the importance of digestive health, we now understand how critical diet is.

Although they often contain good advice, those books only tell readers *what* is happening in the body. With our new understanding of microglia, now we know *why*. Knowing why changes everything. If we don't know why, then our best efforts to treat what is happening are little more than a guessing game.

When it comes to treating pain and depression, this is especially true, since we do not have biomarkers to tell us exactly how much pain patients are in or how far their depression has progressed. We have to take patients' word for it when they say they're in pain; we have little else to go on. Even knowing this, some doctors habitually refuse to believe their patients. When they come to my clinic, patients constantly tell me about doctors who have dismissed or even scorned their symptoms.

Considering how poorly we have understood the nature of pain and depression, this is breathtaking hubris. As I pointed out in Chapter 6, we don't even have a good definition of what disease is. Until now, pain and depression have been far more elusive. With so little information to go on, it's astonishing that a doctor would dare to assume that a patient was wrong about his or her own symptoms.

One of the more outrageous examples of this was with Julie, a 35-year-old patient who came to my office with signs of a stroke. She had difficulty speaking, and the muscles on the right side of her face were flacid. I sent her to the hospital, ordered an MRI of her brain, and called in a neurologist. The MRI results came back normal. When the neurologist was unable to find any other abnormal labs, he discharged her from the hospital.

When Julie returned to my office the next day, the entire right side of her face was distorted. The muscles on one side of her mouth and face were clearly impaired. She was unable to speak without severe distortion. When I tested her, the entire right side of her body demonstrated weakness and pain. She had marked nystagmus, a condition of rapid, involuntary eye movements. All of these things were clear signs of a brain stem stroke.

Alarmed, I asked, "What did the neurologist say?"

Julie struggled to answer. Her speech was garbled, but I could make out the words "He said I should see a psychologist and speech therapist."

I immediately called the neurologist. He explained that all her tests were normal, so there was nothing more he could do. "Clearly, Julie is not normal," I insisted. "Don't you think she needs a further workup?"

Even presented with such conspicuous symptoms, the neurologist was dismissive. He was at the limit of his ability to test and didn't want anything more to do with it. I referred Julie to another neurologist at Georgetown. Eventually, she was diagnosed with a rare neuroinflammatory disease.

Redefining chronic pain, depression, and other neuropsychiatric diseases as neuroinflammatory diseases changes the questions we ask and provides us with the possibility of solutions to these conditions. As we pursue more research in this area, it will also provide us with better testing and treatments.

A new age is dawning for those suffering with chronic pain and depression. The practice of treating the symptoms is coming to an end.

Now that we understand the physiology, we can begin to treat the cause. Understanding the physiology, the divisions between psychiatry and medicine begin to break down. Understanding the physiology allows us to treat people, not labels. If chronic pain and neuropsychiatric conditions share a similar physiology, then our treatments must be all-inclusive, not either-or.

When a young man is suicidally depressed and not responding to conventional psychiatric care, we need to ask more questions. Could he have Lyme disease, biotoxicity disorder, or undiagnosed celiac disease? Has his history of infections and traumas built up and overwhelmed his body?

The reality is that we cannot help everyone. There is still much we have to learn about the neurophysiology of pain and depression. Understanding the physiology of inflammation in the central nervous system is certainly one of the keys. Understanding microglia physiology is at the center of this new understanding, but it is just the beginning. The brain is a vast complex organ. We have spent a century studying neurons, and only recently have we begun to understand the role of the glia cells, the other half of the brain.

Labeling a thing is not knowing it. More than 100 million people in the United States alone live with the labels of chronic pain, depression, PTSD, migraines, fibromyalgia, and anxiety disorders. It is time we stop giving labels based on symptoms and talk about diagnosis based on our understanding of the physiology.

The science is evolving rapidly. Our job as physicians is to bring this new understanding of the physiology into the clinic as quickly as possible. As a patient, your job is to demand a better, more comprehensive medical care system—a system in which your physician is not penalized for spending time with you and rewarded for doing more procedures on you, a system that respects the complexity of your conditions and sees you as an integrated whole.

You need to do your part. You need to be fully active participants in your medical care. Ask questions, do your own research, and, like it or not, eat your vegetables. Pay attention to your diet. Meditate. Exercise. Get proper sleep. Take care of yourself.

When these things happen, there is not only the possibility but indeed the probability of total recovery.

Resources

FINDING A DOCTOR

The leading medical organizations are among the best places to find a medical practitioner in your area. Although some of these physicians will have overlapping skills and specialties, their Web sites will give you a good place to start.

Only a handful of doctors in the country have clinics with a team of specialists, as we do at the Kaplan Center, but you may be able to find an integrative physician—trained in both conventional and alternative medical approaches—who is willing to oversee and coordinate all the elements of treatments with other specialists.

On my Web site (www.kaplanclinic.com), you'll find a useful guide on 18 things to know before selecting a doctor. Among the questions you should ask:

- Is the doctor a legitimate expert?
- Does the doctor try to find the underlying cause or treat the symptoms?
- Does the doctor understand the value of noninvasive manual therapies?
- Is the doctor quick to suggest surgery?
- Is the doctor looking for potential hormonal imbalances?
- Does the doctor consider the importance of nutrition?
- Is the doctor open to working with or leading a team of experts?

Ideally, you will find a family physician or internist with a strong background in integrative medicine. All of the medical schools with integrative medicine training programs have clinics.

Start with Your Team Leader

Complicated conditions can benefit from a variety of treatments. We want to treat the whole body, not its component parts. The best way to do that is to work with a team of experts. Your primary physician will be the leader of that team, consulting with each member of the team and helping to coordinate their treatments.

The organizations below have lists of physicians who already have an integrative orientation. They are well trained in the comprehensive care methods of conventional medicine, but are also open-minded and knowledgeable about alternative approaches. Contact these organizations first for referrals to doctors in your area, then interview several, if you can, before choosing the one who is the best fit.

Consortium of Academic Health Centers for Integrative Medicine
(a comprehensive list of all the integrative health centers in the country)
www.ncbi.nlm.nih.gov/books/NBK83797

American Association of Naturopathic Physicians
www.naturopathic.org

American Holistic Medical Association
www.holisticmedicine.org

Institute for Functional Medicine
www.functionalmedicine.org

American College for Advancement of Medicine
www.acamnet.org

Team Members: Specialized Treatments

Once you've chosen a primary physician to partner with in your recovery, some of these specialized treatments may be appropriate. These organizations are reliable sources of referrals in each of the categories.

Musculoskeletal Medicine

For realigning the body; restoring normal structural integrity and function to the muscles, bones, and organs; minimizing the risk of injury; and improving health.

American Academy of Osteopathy
https://netforum.avectra.com/eweb/StartPage.aspx?Site=AAO

American Chiropractic Association
www.acatoday.org

Prolotherapy Treatment

For muscular and joint pain, particularly if it has not responded to treatment. It can restore structural integrity.

Hackett Hemwall Foundation
www.hacketthemwall.org

American Association of Orthopaedic Medicine
www.aaomed.org

Acupuncture Treatment

For a wide range of conditions, including acute injuries, emotional and physical traumas, and strengthening of the body systems. It reduces inflammation and pain by enlisting the body's natural opioid system.

American Academy of Medical Acupuncture
(medical physicians who practice acupuncture)
www.medicalacupuncture.org

American Association of Acupuncture and Oriental Medicine
(acupuncturists who are not physicians)
www.aaaomonline.org

Biotoxicity Treatment

For testing and evaluation of Lyme disease and related tick-borne diseases, as well as environmental toxins.

American College for Advancement in Medicine
www.acam.org

American Academy of Environmental Medicine
http://aaemonline.org

GETTING THE RIGHT TESTS

If you were my patient, I would evaluate your condition with a host of tests. You will find that many integrative medicine doctors take a similar approach. The tests below are not always included.

These are tests that can easily be obtained by your family physician or internist, but you may have to request them. If you suspect these tests may be relevant for you, do not hesitate to consult your doctor about them. If you are met with reluctance, it may be useful to explain that, since your symptoms have not yet been alleviated, these are tests you would like to use to explore and potentially eliminate possible causes of your condition.

Gluten Intolerance/Celiac Disease Tests

Any standard medical laboratory can do these tests. The appropriate test checks for IgG antigliadin antibodies, IgA antiendomysial antibodies, and tissue transglutaminase antibodies (tTG) in blood, as well as stool antigliadin (IgA and tTG).[1] We know the genetic markers for celiac disease but not for gluten intolerance. The only true way to test for gluten sensitivity is to eliminate it from your diet for 6 weeks and see if you feel better. Often patients who do have gluten sensitivity find that their brain fog disappears and their sinus congestion subsides. It is an experiment you can easily try yourself. Be sure to read food labels. Various forms of wheat are included in a lot of packaged goods. Oddly enough, gluten can also be found in shampoo, toothpaste, and cosmetics, but you are unlikely to be affected by those small amounts unless you have celiac disease.

The genetic tests for celiac cannot confirm that you have it. As many as 35 percent of the population have a genetic proclivity for celiac disease, but only 3 percent actually develop the disease. If the tests show that you are among those at risk for celiac, it is best to avoid gluten as a precaution. It may minimize your chances of getting it. The typical age of onset for celiac disease is 40 to 60 years old.

Lyme Disease

Many of my patients who have Lyme disease do not remember being bitten by a tick. It is an infectious disease that clearly upregulates microglia. It is easy to miss and difficult to diagnose. There is also a lot of controversy about treating it. If you suspect that you have Lyme disease, it makes sense to be tested, even if you never saw the tick.

Although the symptoms of Lyme disease can be mistaken for other conditions, a patient with Lyme feels very sick. The disease can start with what seems to be the flu, but is then followed by a chronic neck ache unexplained by accident or trauma. The patient may have digestive problems, headaches, significant fatigue, or night sweats. The most common symptom is joint pain that moves around the body (migrating arthralgia).

An excellent guide to this disease is Richard Horowitz's book, *Why Can't I Get Better? Solving the Mystery of Lyme & Chronic Disease* (St. Martin's Press, 2013). For details on testing, contact the International Lyme and Associated Diseases Society (www.ilads.org).

Chronic Epstein-Barr Virus

This condition creates an inflammatory state that manifests as chronic fatigue. Patients with this condition are not simply tired, like healthy people feel when they don't get enough sleep or good nutrition; they feel so sick that it impairs their ability to function in the simplest daily tasks. They have difficulty concentrating or doing things they could ordinarily do without a problem.

The condition is often overlooked or attributed to other things, but missing this diagnosis is unnecessary, since good testing is available. We follow a testing and treatment protocol published by researchers at Stanford University, who use IFA testing to make a diagnosis.[2] The only lab using this protocol is Quest Diagnostics.

For details on testing, you can contact Quest Diagnostics (www.questdiagnostics.com).

Biotoxicity

Ritchie Shoemaker, MD, discovered the markers for biotoxicity from indoor mold and other biotoxins, such as those associated with heavy metals, spider bites, and Lyme disease. He has developed a quick early-screening test, as well as a treatment for the condition. Biotoxins are poisonings that occur as a result of exposure to certain environmental toxins. Although the symptoms vary, making it hard to diagnose, they can include transitory numbness in arms and legs, depression, emotional instability, fatigue, brain fog, skin rashes, asthma, and breathing problems.

Dr. Shoemaker's book *Surviving Mold Life in the Era of Dangerous Building* (Otter Bay Books, 2011) provides an insightful reference. His Web site, www.chronicneurotoxins.com, contains an early-screening test for biotoxicity of all kinds, called Visual Contrast Sensitivity, that can be taken online.

Sleep Disorders

Whether you snore or wake up tired in the mornings, if you have any reason to suspect that you are not getting restful sleep for medical reasons, it's important to have it checked. Inadequate rest and hypoxia can take years off of your life.

For the industry standard for early screening of a sleep disorder:

Epworth Sleepiness Scale Quiz
www.stanford.edu/~dement/epworth.html

For a sleep laboratory evaluation and/or overnight testing:

American Academy of Sleep Medicine
www.aasmnet.org

For a reliable home testing device called WatchPAT:

Itamar Medical
www.itamar-medical.com/WatchPAT/Patient.html

Thyroid Balance

Because so many patients have an imbalance in the hypothalamic pituitary axis, I regularly include a thyroid test. Thyroid function can be adversely affected by medications (such as opioids, lithium, and some antiseizure medications), high doses of the isoflavonoids (phytoestrogens) found in soy products, as well as environmental toxins (such as pesticides and bisphenol A, the resin used to coat food cans). Testosterone, lithium, and beta-blockers can create hyperthyroidism.

Healthy thyroid hormones are vital for the regeneration of neurons in the brain, as well as metabolic functions in the body. Treatment and diagnosis for hypothyroidism can be controversial. Most conventional physicians will tell you only the TSH and T4 need to be measured. In my experience, TSH, at a minimum, and the free forms of T3 and T4 need to be measured. The normal values vary by the patient's age and norms used by the lab. Keep in mind that your own normative value may not match the value set by the lab.

The lower limit may not be right for you, but that is of less concern, since you can take thyroid supplements. However, you do not want to exceed the upper limits of free T3 or T4 set by the lab. T4 is the predominant hormone produced by the gland. T3 is produced in the tissues by converting T4 to T3. You can have a T3 deficiency even if your tests show a normal TSH and a normal T4. If the enzyme needed to convert T4 to T3 is ineffective, your T3 may be low regardless. That's why all three tests need to be done.

Testing for bound versions of the hormone is standard testing procedure, but I have found that free versions are more revealing, even if they are controversial. I highly recommend Mary Shomon's *Living Well with Hypothyroidism* (HarperResource, 2005).

ENDNOTES

INTRODUCTION

1 Gary Wolf, "Steve Jobs: The Next Insanely Great Thing," *Wired*, April 2002, accessed October 2013, www.wired.com/wired/archive/4.02/jobs_pr.html.

2 *The Profession of Physical Therapy*, Jones & Bartlett Learning, accessed October 2012, http://samples.jbpub.com/9780763781309/81309_CH01_FINAL.pdf.

3 James Reston, "Now, About My Operation in Peking," *New York Times*, July 26, 1971, http://graphics8.nytimes.com/packages/pdf/health/1971acupuncture.pdf.

4 Ibid.

5 Ibid.

6 Ibid.

7 "PET scan," MedlinePlus, last modified November 9, 2012, www.nlm.nih.gov/medlineplus/ency/article/003827.htm.

8 "Barry Marshall, M.D.: The Courage to Experiment," interview, Academy of Achievement, May 23, 1998, last modified September 23, 2010, www.achievement.org/autodoc/page/mar1int-3.

9 "The Interview Archive: Barry Marshall, Scientist," BBC World Service, November 6, 2010, accessed October 2012, www.bbc.co.uk/programmes/p00bqtff.

10 David M. Eisenberg et al., "Unconventional Medicine in the United States—Prevalence, Costs, and Patterns of Use," *New England Journal of Medicine* 328, no. 4 (January 28, 1993): 246–52.

11 Ibid.

12 Ibid.

13 Ibid.

14 Bill Hall and Anita Greene, "NIH Panel Issues Consensus Statement on Acupuncture," NIH News Release, November 5, 1997, accessed October 2012, www.nih.gov/news/pr/nov97/od-05.htm.

15 Eisenberg et al., "Unconventional Medicine."

16 Ibid.

17 "NIH Consensus Development Program," National Institutes of Health, accessed October 2012, http://prevention.nih.gov/cdp/faq.aspx#whatistheCDP.

CHAPTER 1

1 Andrew Walsh, "The Musket: Use in Battle and a Dreadful Injury," *Tudor Stuff: Tudor History from the Heart of England* (blog), September 25, 2009, http://tudor stuff.wordpress.com/2009/09/25/the-musket-use-in-battle-a-dreadful-injury.

2 Free Dictionary by Farlex, Medical Dictionary, s.v. "causalgia," accessed October 2012, http://medical-dictionary.thefreedictionary.com/causalgia.

3 "Phantom Limb and Causalgia: The Tragic Enigmas," Louise M. Darling Biomedical Library, UCLA, 1998, accessed November 2012, http://unitproj.library.ucla.edu/biomed/his/painexhibit/panel4.htm.

4 Victor Kuenkel, "Causalgia—Pathogenesis and Treatment," *California Medicine* 77, no. 6 (December 1952): 374–76, www.ncbi.nlm.nih.gov/pmc/articles/PMC1521551.

5 "Complex Regional Pain Syndrome Fact Sheet," National Institute of Neurological Disorders and Stroke, NIH Publication No. 13-4173, last modified July 12, 2013, www.ninds.nih.gov/disorders/reflex_sympathetic_dystrophy/detail_reflex_sympathetic_dystrophy.htm.

6 Ibid.

7 "Conditions Treated: Causalgia," UCLA Neurosurgery, accessed November 2012, http://neurosurgery.ucla.edu/body.cfm?id=1123&ref=18&action=detail.

8 "Complex Regional Pain Syndrome Fact Sheet."

9 "Phantom Limb and Causalgia."

10 "Complex Regional Pain Syndrome Fact Sheet."

11 "Phantom Limb and Causalgia."

12 "Complex Regional Pain Syndrome Fact Sheet."

13 "Phantom Limb and Causalgia."

14 Joe Fahy, "Too Young for Pain," *Pittsburgh Post-Gazette*, October 5, 2005, www.post-gazette.com/stories/news/health/too-young-for-pain-603546/.

15 Childhood RND Educational Foundation, http://www.childhoodrnd.org.

16 Fahy, "Too Young for Pain."

17 "A Servant to Servants," line 58, from *The Poetry of Robert Frost* (New York: Holt, Rinehart and Winston,1969), 64.

18 Fahy, "Too Young for Pain."

19 Institute of Medicine Report from the Committee on Advancing Pain Research, Care, and Education, *Relieving Pain in America: A Blueprint for Transforming Prevention, Care, Education, and Research* (Washington, DC: The National Academies Press, 2011), http://books.nap.edu/openbook.php?record_id=13172&page=1.

20 "Biography" of Norm Shealy, sHEALy Wellness, accessed October 2012, www.normshealy.com/biography.

21 Brit Brogaard, DMSci, PhD, "The Chemistry of Emotional Pain," Lovesick Love, April 3, 2011, accessed November 2012, www.lovesicklove.com/2011/04/the-chemistry-of-emotional-pain.html.

22 Brogaard, "The Chemistry of Emotional Pain."

23 A. Dray, "Inflammatory Mediators of Pain," *British Journal of Anaesthesia* 75 (1995): 125–31, http://bja.oxfordjournals.org/content/75/2/125.full.pdf.

24 I. D. Grachev, B. E. Fredrickson, and A. V. Apkarian, "Abnormal Brain Chemistry in Chronic Back Pain: An In Vivo Proton Magnetic Resonance Spectroscopy Study," *Pain* 89, no. 1 (December 15, 2000): 7–18, www.painjournalonline.com/article/S0304-3959%2800%2900340-7/abstract.

25 Michael Specter, "Rethinking the Brain: How the Songs of Canaries Upset a Fundamental Principle of Science," *New Yorker*, July 23, 2001, https://www.msu.edu/course/psy/401/snapshot.afs/Readings/WK6.Supplement%20-%20New%20Yorker%20Article.pdf.

26 "Definition of Chronic Pain," MedicineNet.com, accessed September 20, 2012, www.medterms.com/script/main/art.asp?articlekey=22430.

27 H. Merskey, N. Bogduk, eds., "Part III: Pain Terms—A Current List with Definitions and Notes on Usage," in *Classification of Chronic Pain*, 2nd ed., IASP Task Force on Taxonomy (Seattle: IASP Press, 1994): 209, www.iasp-pain.org/AM/Template.cfm?Section=Pain_Definitions.

28 Dennis Turk, "Assess the Person, Not Just the Pain," *Pain: Clinical Updates* 1, no. 3 (September 1993), www.iasp-pain.org/AM/AMTemplate.cfm?Section=Pain_Definitions&SECTION=Pain_Definitions&CONTENTID=7627&TEMPLATE=/CM/ContentDisplay.cfm.

29 Robert Louis Stevenson, *A Child's Garden of Verses* (New York: Charles Scribner's Sons, 1931), 18.

30 27.2 percent of people older than 26 years had osteoarthritis. Over age 60, 37.4 percent had osteoarthritis. Of all those who had it, only 12.1 percent had symptoms.

31 Jane Gross, "Some Veterans Fear Reopening Psychic Wounds," *New York Times*, March 20, 1991, www.nytimes.com/1991/03/20/us/some-veterans-fear-reopening-psychic-wounds.html.

32 Kurt C. Stange, "The Problem of Fragmentation and the Need for Integrative Solutions," *Annals of Family Medicine* 7, no. 2 (March 2009): 100–103, www.ncbi.nlm.nih.gov/pmc/articles/PMC2653966/.

33 Ibid.

34 Stuart Firestein, *Ignorance: How It Drives Science* (New York: Oxford University Press, 2012), 17.

35 Jonah Lehrer, "The Reinvention of the Self: Brain and Behavior," *Seed Magazine*, February 22, 2006, http://seedmagazine.com/content/article/the_reinvention_of_the_self.

36 Richard J. Clofine, "Respiratory-Circulatory Method of Zink," Aumdoc Osteopathic Medicine, accessed August 2013, www.aumdoc.com/events/respcirc.htm.

37 Ibid.

38 William I. B. Beveridge, *The Art of Scientific Investigation* (Caldwell, NJ: Blackburn Press, 2004), 32.

39 R. Shoemaker and D. House, "A Time-Series Study of Sick Building Syndrome: Chronic, Biotoxin-Associated Illness from Exposure to Water-Damaged Buildings," Neurotoxicology and Teratology 27, no. 1 (January–February 2005): 29–46, www.ncbi.nlm.nih.gov/pubmed/15681119.

40 "What Is Osteopathic Medicine?" American Association of Colleges of Osteopathic Medicine, accessed November 2013, www.aacom.org/about/osteomed/Pages/default.aspx.

41 Ibid.

42 Biology Online, s.v. "punctum caecum," accessed October 2012, www.biology-online.org/dictionary/Punctum_caecum.

43 "Speed of the Earth's Rotation," NASA Goddard Space Flight Center, Ask an Astrophysicist, last updated December 1, 2012, http://imagine.gsfc.nasa.gov/docs/ask_astro/answers/970401c.html.

44 Christopher Chabris and Daniel Simons, *The Invisible Gorilla: How Our Intuitions Deceive Us* (New York: MJF Books, 2012), 6.

45 Ritchie C. Shoemaker with Patti Schmidt, *Mold Warriors: Fighting America's Hidden Health Threat* (Baltimore: Otter Bay Books, 2010), 7.

46 Beveridge, *The Art of Scientific Investigation*, 36.

CHAPTER 2

1 Gwenn Herman and Mary French, *Making the Invisible Visible: Chronic Pain Manual for Health Care Providers* (Potomac, MD: Pain Connection, 2009) www.painconnection.org/updates/painbook.html.

2 C. Brock et al., "Opioid-Induced Bowel Dysfunction: Pathophysiology and Management," *Drugs* 72, no. 14 (October 1, 2012): 1847–65, www.ncbi.nlm.nih.gov/pubmed/22950533.

3 S. Prakash et al., "Gut Microbiota: Next Frontier in Understanding Human Health and Development of Biotherapeutics," *Biologics* 5 (2011): 71–86, www.ncbi.nlm.nih.gov/pmc/articles/PMC3156250.

4 A. Risser et al., "NSAID Prescribing Precautions," *American Family Physician* 80, no. 12 (December 15, 2009): 1371–78, www.ncbi.nlm.nih.gov/pubmed/20000300.

5 D. Adebayo and I. Bjarnason, "Is Non-Steroidal Anti-Inflamma[t]ory Drug (NSAID) Enteropathy Clinically More Important Than NSAID Gastropathy?" *Postgraduate Medical Journal* 82, no. 965 (March 2006): 186–91, www.ncbi.nlm.nih.gov/pmc/articles/PMC2563708.

6 Elizabeth Lipski, *Digestive Wellness: How to Strengthen the Immune System and Prevent Disease Through Healthy Digestion*, 3rd ed. (New York: McGraw-Hill, 2004).

7 W. Supornsilpchai, S. M. le Grand, and A. Srikiatkhachorn, "Involvement of Pro-Nociceptive 5-HT2A Receptor in the Pathogenesis of Medication-Overuse Headache," *Headache* 50, no. 2 (February 2010): 185–97, www.ncbi.nlm.nih.gov/pubmed/20039957.

8 S. J. Tepper, "Medication-Overuse Headache," *Continuum* 18, no. 4 (August 2012): 807–22, www.ncbi.nlm.nih.gov/pubmed/22868543.

9 D. F. Kripke, R. D. Langer, and L. E. Kline, "Hypnotics' Association with Mortality or Cancer: A Matched Cohort Study," Abstract, *BMJ Open* 2, no. 1 (February 27, 2012), http://bmjopen.bmj.com/content/2/1/e000850.abstract.

10 Hartmut Schulz, "Rethinking Sleep Analysis: Comment on the AASM Manual for the Scoring of Sleep and Associated Events," *Journal of Clinical Sleep Medicine* 4, no. 2 (April 2008): 99–103, www.ncbi.nlm.nih.gov/pmc/articles/PMC2335403. The 1968 Rechtschaffen and Kales standardization of four stages of NREM sleep was revised by the American Academy of Sleep Medicine in 2007, reducing four stages to three.

11 "What Happens When You Sleep?" National Sleep Foundation, accessed February 2013, www.sleepfoundation.org/article/how-sleep-works/what-happens-when-you-sleep.

12 Healthy Sleep Glossary, Harvard University, accessed February 2013, http://healthysleep.med.harvard.edu/glossary/n-p.

13 "What Happens When You Sleep?"

14 Edward B. Blanchard and Edward J. Hickling, *After the Crash: Psychological Assessment and Treatment of Survivors of Motor Vehicle Accidents*, 2nd ed. (American Psychological Association, 2003), www.apa.org/pubs/books/4317028.aspx.

15 J. G. Beck and S. F. Coffey, "Assessment and Treatment of PTSD after a Motor Vehicle Collision: Empirical Findings and Clinical Observations," *Professional Psychology, Research and Practice* 38, no. 6 (December 2007): 629–39, www.ncbi.nlm.nih.gov/pmc/articles/PMC2396820.

16 "What Is Prolotherapy?" American Osteopathic Association of Prolotherapy Regenerative Medicine, accessed October 2012, www.acopms.com.

17 "Treatment of PTSD," US Department of Veterans Affairs, National Center for PTSD, www.ptsd.va.gov/public/pages/treatment-ptsd.asp.

CHAPTER 3

1 "Tailbone (Coccyx) Injury," WebMD, accessed October 2012, www.webmd.com/fitness-exercise/tailbone-coccyx-injury.

2 Virginia P. Wilson, "Janet G. Travell, MD: A Daughter's Recollection," *Texas Heart Institute Journal* 30, no. 1 (2003): 8–12, www.ncbi.nlm.nih.gov/pmc/articles/PMC152828.

3 "What Is Myofascia?" Jenings Training and Treatment Centre, accessed December 2012, http://jenings.com/what-is-fascia.html.

4 Eileen DiGiovanna, Stanley Schiowitz, and Dennis J. Dowling, "Myofascial (Soft Tissue) Techniques," chapter 12 in *An Osteopathic Approach to Diagnosis and Treatment*, 3rd ed. (Philadelphia: Lippincott Williams & Wilkins, 2005).

5 Burton Schuler, "Dr. Janet Travell: JFK, Your Feet and Trigger Points Explained by a Podiatrist," Foot Care for You, accessed January 2013, www.footcare4u.com/category/foot-ailments-treatments/common-foot-ailments/mortons-toe/resources/dr-janet-travell.

6 E. A. Tough et al., "Variability of Criteria Used to Diagnose Myofascial Trigger Point Pain Syndrome—Evidence from a Review of the Literature," *Clinical Journal of Pain* 23, no. 3 (March–April 2007): 278–86, www.ncbi.nlm.nih.gov/pubmed/17314589.

7 Marek Jantos, "Understanding Chronic Pelvic Pain," *Pelviperineology* 26, no. 2 (June 2007): 66–69, www.pelviperineology.org/practical/chronic_pelvic_pain.html.

8 Ibid.

9 American Association of Colleges of Osteopathic Medicine, *Glossary of Osteopathic Terminology*, 2012, 28.

10 DiGiovanna, Schiowitz, and Dowling, *An Osteopathic Approach*, 80–82.

11 Janet G. Travell and David G. Simons, *Myofascial Pain and Dysfunction: The Trigger Point Manual: Volume 2, The Lower Extremities* (Baltimore: Williams & Wilkins, 1992).

12 R. K. Hofbauer, H. W. Olausson, and M. C. Bushnell, "Thermal and Tactile Sensory Deficits and Allodynia in a Nerve-Injured Patient: A Multimodal Psychophysical and Functional Magnetic Resonance Imaging Study," *Clinical Journal of Pain* 22, no. 1 (January 2006): 104–8; R. C. Coghill et al., "Pain Intensity Processing within the Human Brain: A Bilateral, Distributed Mechanism," *Journal of Neurophysiology* 82, no. 4 (October 1999): 1934–43; and C. L. McGrath et al., "Toward a Neuroimaging Treatment Selection Biomarker for Major Depressive Disorder," *JAMA Psychiatry* 70, no. 8 (August 2013): 821–29.

13 B. A. Arnow et al., "Comorbid Depression, Chronic Pain and Disability in Primary Care," *Psychosomatic Medicine* 68, no. 2 (March–April 2006): 262–8; and W. M. Compton et al., "Changes in the Prevalence of Major Depression and Comorbid Substance Use Disorders in the United States between 1991–1992 and 2001–2002," *American Journal of Psychiatry* 163, no. 12 (December 2006): 2141–47.

14 Siegfried Mense, David G. Simons, and I. Jon Russell, *Muscle Pain: Understanding Its Nature, Diagnosis, and Treatment* (Philadelphia: Lippincott Williams & Wilkins, 2001), 121.

15 Harold Merskey and Nikolai Bogduck, eds., "Pain Terms, a Current List with Definitions and Notes on Usage," part III in *Classification of Chronic Pain*, 2nd ed. (Seattle: IASP Press, 1994), 209–214.

16 Arnow et al., "Comorbid Depression, Chronic Pain and Disability," 262–68.

17 John F. Steege, "Basic Philosophy of the Integrated Approach: Overcoming the Mind-Body Split," in *Chronic Pelvic Pain: An Integrated Approach*, ed. by John F. Steege, Deborah A. Metzger, and Barbara S. Levy (Philadelphia: Saunders, 1998), 6–12.

18 John E. Sarno, *Healing Back Pain: The Mind-Body Connection* (New York: Warner Books, 1991), 1.

19 Ibid., 2.

20 B. Nicholson, "Responsible Prescribing of Opioids for the Management of Chronic Pain," *Drugs* 63, no. 1 (2003): 17–32, www.ncbi.nlm.nih.gov/pubmed/12487620.

21 B. Bannwarth, "Risk-Benefit Assessment of Opioids in Chronic Noncancer Pain," *Drug Safety* 21, no. 4 (October 1999): 283–96, www.ncbi.nlm.nih.gov/pubmed/10514020.

CHAPTER 4

1 "Multiple Sclerosis," *A.D.A.M. Medical Encyclopedia*, PubMed Health, accessed April 2013, www.ncbi.nlm.nih.gov/pubmedhealth/PMH0001747.

2 "Post-Treatment Lyme Disease Syndrome," Centers for Disease Control and Prevention, www.cdc.gov/lyme/postLDS.

3 K. Berndtson, "Review of Evidence for Immune Evasion and Persistent Infection in Lyme Disease," *International Journal of General Medicine* 6 (2013): 291–306, published online April 23, 2013, www.ncbi.nlm.nih.gov/pmc/articles/PMC3636972.

4 W. M. Compton et al., "Changes in the Prevalence of Major Depression and Comorbid Substance Use Disorders in the United States between 1991–1992 and 2001–2002," *American Journal of Psychiatry* 163, no. 12 (December 2006): 2141–47; B. A. Arnow et al., "Comorbid Depression, Chronic Pain and Disability in Primary Care," *Psychosomatic Medicine* 68, no. 2 (March–April 2006): 262–68; and R. C. Kessler, K. R. Merikangas, and P. S. Wang, "Prevalence, Comorbidity, and Service Utilization for Mood Disorders in the United States at the Beginning of the Twenty-First Century," *Annual Review of Clinical Psychology* 3 (2007): 137–158.

5 M. J. Bair et al., "Impact of Pain on Depression Treatment Response in Primary Care," *Psychosomatic Medicine* 66, no. 1 (January–February 2004): 17–22, www.ncbi.nlm.nih.gov/pubmed/14747633.

6 M. J. Robinson et al., "Depression and Pain," *Frontiers in Bioscience* 14 (June 1, 2009): 5031–51, www.bioscience.org/2009/v14/af/3585/fulltext.htm.

7 R. Douglas Fields, *The Other Brain* (New York: Simon and Schuster, 2010), http://theotherbrainbook.com.

8 P. Amodio et al., "Mood, Cognition and EEG Changes during Interferon Alpha (Alpha-IFN) Treatment for Chronic Hepatitis C," *Journal of Affective Disorders* 84, no. 1 (January 2005): 93–98; and A. D. Valentine and C.A. Meyers, "Neurobehavioral Effects of Interferon Therapy," *Current Psychiatry Reports* 7, no. 5 (October 2005): 391–95.

9 M. Catena-Dell'Osso et al., "Inflammatory and Neurodegenerative Pathways in Depression: A New Avenue for Antidepressant Development?" *Current Medicinal Chemistry* 18, no. 2 (2011): 245–55; and K. A. Jones and C. Thomsen, "The Role of the Innate Immune System in Psychiatric Disorders," *Molecular and Cellular Neurosciences* 53 (March 2013): 52–62.

10 M. E. Robinson et al., "Gray Matter Volumes of Pain-Related Brain Areas Are Decreased in Fibromyalgia Syndrome," *Journal of Pain* 12, no. 4 (April 2011): 436–43; H. A. Jurgens and R. W. Johnson, "Dysregulated Neuronal-Microglial Cross-Talk during Aging, Stress and Inflammation," *Experimental Neurology* 233, no. 1 (January 2012): 40–48; S. Amor et al., "Inflammation in Neurodegenerative Diseases," *Immunology* 129, no. 2 (February 2010): 154–169; and S. H. Fatemi et al., "Consensus Paper: Pathological Role of the Cerebellum in Autism," *Cerebellum* 11, no. 3 (September 2012): 777–807.

11 C. J. Woolf, "Central Sensitization: Implications for the Diagnosis and Treatment of Pain," supplement, *Pain* 152, no. S3 (March 2011): S2–S15, www.ncbi.nlm.nih.gov/pubmed/20961685.

12 Fields, *The Other Brain*.

13 J. A. McClain et al., "Adolescent Binge Alcohol Exposure Induces Long-Lasting Partial Activation of Microglia," *Brain, Behavior, and Immunity* 25, no. S1 (June 2011): S120–S128, www.ncbi.nlm.nih.gov/pubmed/21262339.

14 Jonah Lehrer, "The Reinvention of the Self: Brain and Behavior," Seed Magazine, February 22, 2006, 1, http://seedmagazine.com/content/article/the_reinvention_of_the_self/?page=all&p=y.

15 William I. B. Beveridge, *The Art of Scientific Investigation* (Caldwell, NJ: Blackburn Press, 2004).

16 Ibid.

17 Sarah Boseley, "Obama Unveils Brain Mapping Initiative and Calls for Further Research," *Guardian* April 2, 2013, www.theguardian.com/science/2013/apr/02/obama-brain-initiative-fight-disease.

18 Human Brain Project, www.humanbrainproject.eu.

19 R. Douglas Fields, "Beyond the Neuron Doctrine," *Scientific American*, June 2006, 21–27.

20 Philip M. Boffey, "The Next Frontier Is Inside Your Brain," *New York Times*, February 23, 2013, www.nytimes.com/2013/02/24/opinion/sunday/the-next-frontier-is-in-your-brain.html?_r=0.

21 C. L. Dolman in *Textbook of Neuropathology*, edited by R. L. Davis and D. M. Robertson (Williams & Wilkins: Baltimore, 1991), 141–63.

22 Fields, *The Other Brain*.

23 R. Douglas Fields, "The New Brain: How Your Brain and Our Understanding of It Are Constantly Changing," *Psychology Today*, December 15, 2009, www.psychologytoday.com/blog/the-new-brain/200912/glia-the-other-brain.

24 "Fibromyalgia," National Institute of Arthritis and Musculoskeletal and Skin Diseases, NIH Publication 12-5326, August 2012, www.niams.nih.gov/health_info/Fibromyalgia.

CHAPTER 5

1 These descriptions come from two excellent resources: Elizabeth Lipski, *Digestive Wellness: How to Strengthen the Immune System and Prevent Disease through Healthy Digestion*, 3rd ed. (New York: McGraw-Hill, 2004); and "Your Digestive System and How It Works," National Digestive Diseases Information Clearinghouse, NIH Publication No. 08-2681, last updated April 23, 2012, http://digestive.niddk.nih.gov/ddiseases/pubs/yrdd.

2 Adam Hadhazy, "Think Twice: How the Gut's 'Second Brain' Influences Mood and Well-Being," *Scientific American*, February 24, 2010, www.scientificamerican.com/article.cfm?id=gut-second-brain.

3 Michael D. Gershon, MD, *The Second Brain* (New York, HarperCollins, 1998).

4 Lipski, *Digestive Wellness*.

5 Hadhazy, "Think Twice."

6 Ibid.

7 Ibid.

8 Ibid.

9 Lipski, *Digestive Wellness*.

10 Ibid.

11 Ibid.

12 Ibid.

13 Carlo M. Cipolla, "A Plague Doctor," in *The Medieval City*, edited by Harry A. Miskimin, David Herlihy, and A. L. Udovitch (New Haven, CT: Yale University Press, 1977).

14 Lipski, *Digestive Wellness*.

15 Ibid.

16 Ibid.

17 Ibid.

18 Ibid.

19 Ibid.

20 Michael Greger, MD, "SAD States: Standard American Diet State-by-State Comparison," NutritionFacts.org, May 22, 2012, http://nutritionfacts.org/video/sad-states-standard-american-diet-state-by-state-comparison.

21 Lipski, *Digestive Wellness*.

22 Ibid.

23 Ibid.

24 D. Kiefer and L. Ali-Akbarian, "A Brief Evidence-Based Review of Two Gastrointestinal Illnesses: Irritable Bowel and Leaky Gut Syndromes," *Alternative Therapies in Health and Medicine* 10, no. 3 (May–June 2004): 22–30; quiz 31, 92.

25 "Pioneering Researcher Alessio Fasano MD on Gluten, Autoimmunity & Leaky Gut," interview by Chris Kresser, *Revolution Health Radio*, August 8, 2012, http://chriskresser.com/pioneering-researcher-alessio-fasano-m-d-on-gluten-autoimmunity-leaky-gut.

26 Lipski, *Digestive Wellness*.

27 Ibid.

28 A. Fasano, "Zonulin and Its Regulation of Intestinal Barrier Function: The Biological Door to Inflammation, Autoimmunity, and Cancer," *Physiological Review* 91, no. 1 (January 2011): 151–75, www.ncbi.nlm.nih.gov/pubmed/21248165.

29 Ibid.

30 Ibid.

31 A. Fasano et al., "Prevalence of Celiac Disease in At-Risk and Not-At-Risk Groups in the United States," *Archives of Internal Medicine* 163, no. 3 (February 20, 2003): 286–92, www.ncbi.nlm.nih.gov/pubmed/12578508.

32 Melinda Beck, "Clues to Gluten Sensitivity," *Wall Street Journal*, March 15, 2011, http://online.wsj.com/news/articles/SB10001424052748704893604576200393522456636.

33 Ibid.

34 Ibid.

35 Ibid.

36 Moises Velasquez-Manoff, "Who Has the Guts for Gluten?" *New York Times*, February 23, 2013, www.nytimes.com/2013/02/24/opinion/sunday/what-really-causes-celiac-disease.html.

37 Ibid.

38 Ibid.

39 Ibid.

40 Ibid.

41 Ibid.

42 Ibid.

CHAPTER 6

1 Claudia Craig Marek, *The First Year: Fibromyalgia—An Essential Guide for the Newly Diagnosed* (New York: Da Capo, 2003), xix.

2 Ibid.

3 Stacey Butterfield, "Fibromyalgia's Symptoms Real but Be Cautious in Diagnosis," American College of Physicians, *ACP Internist*, May 2009, www.acpinternist.org/archives/2009/05/fibromyalgia.htm.

4 Marek, *The First Year: Fibromyalgia.*

5 Butterfield, "Fibromyalgia's Symptoms Real."

6 Marek, *The First Year.*

7 U.S. Food and Drug Administration, "FDA Approves First Drug for Treating Fibromyalgia," news release, June 21, 2007, www.fda.gov/NewsEvents/Newsroom/PressAnnouncements/2007/ucm108936.htm.

8 "Lyrica Oral: Side Effects," WebMD, accessed August 2013, www.webmd.com/drugs/drug-93965-Lyrica+Oral.aspx?drugid=93965&drugname=Lyrica+Oral.

9 J. A. Capitán, J. A. Cuesta, and J. Bascompte, "Species Are to Ecosystems as Cells Are to the Human Body, according to a Mathematical Model Developed at UC3M," *Journal of Theoretical Biology* 269, no. 1 (January 21, 2011): 344–55, www.uc3m.es/portal/page/portal/actualidad_cientifica/noticias/Species_ecosystems.

10 Ibid.

11 "C. Difficile: Symptoms," Mayo Clinic, accessed August 2013, www.mayoclinic.com/health/c-difficile/DS00736/DSECTION=symptoms.

12 J. Z. Goldenberg et al., "Probiotics for the Prevention of Clostridium Difficile–Associated Diarrhea in Adults and Children, *Cochrane Database of Systematic Reviews* 5 (May 31, 2013): CD006095, www.ncbi.nlm.nih.gov/pubmed/23728658.

13 R. K. Rude, "Magnesium Metabolism and Deficiency," *Endocrinology and Metabolism Clinics of North America* 22, no. 2 (June 1993): 377–95, www.ncbi.nlm.nih.gov/pubmed/8325293.

14 C. Feillet-Coudray et al., "Exchangeable Magnesium Pool Masses in Healthy Women: Effects of Magnesium Supplementation," *American Journal of Clinical Nutrition* 75, no. 1 (January 2002): 72–78, www.ncbi.nlm.nih.gov/pubmed/11756062.

15 "Nutrient Intakes," USDA Human Nutrition, last modified July 29, 2009, www.ars.usda.gov/Services/docs.htm?docid=15672.

16 R. K. Rude, "Magnesium Deficiency: A Cause of Heterogeneous Disease in Humans," *Journal of Bone and Mineral Research* 13, no. 4 (April 1998): 749–58.

17 Centers for Disease Control and Prevention, *Laboratory Medicine Best Practices: Developing an Evidence-Based Review and Evaluation Process. Final Technical Report 2007: Phase I* (Atlanta: US Department of Health and Human Services, 2008), www.futurelabmedicine.org/pdfs/Phase%20I%20Final%20report%20LabBestPractice.pdf.

18 "How Reliable Is Laboratory Testing?" Lab Tests Online, American Association for Clinical Chemistry, last modified March 18, 2013, https://labtestsonline.org/understanding/features/reliability/start/1.

19 Ibid.

20 *JAMA: The Journal of the American Medical Association*, accessed May 2013, http://jama.jamanetwork.com/public/InstructionsForAuthors.aspx.

21 Centers for Disease Control and Prevention, *Laboratory Medicine Best Practices.*

22 "How Reliable Is Laboratory Testing?"

23 Jane E. Brody, "Injections to Kick-Start Tissue Repair," *New York Times*, August 7, 2007, www.nytimes.com/2007/08/07/health/07brod.html?_r=0.

24 "Alternative Treatments," *Mayo Clinic Health Letter* 23, no. 4 (April 2005): 3, www.prolotherapy.com/Mayo-Clinic-Prolo%202005.pdf.

25 Laura Johannes, "A Pinch of Sugar for Pain," *Wall Street Journal*, October 19, 2010, http://online.wsj.com/article/SB10001424052702304410504575560214236534310.html.

26 R. J. Engler et al., "Half- vs Full-Dose Trivalent Inactivated Influenza Vaccine (2004–2005): Age, Dose, and Sex Effects on Immune Responses," *Archives of Internal Medicine* 168, no. 22 (December 8, 2008): 2405–14, www.ncbi.nlm.nih.gov/pubmed/19064822.

27 Melinda Wenner Moyer, "Drug Problem: Women Aren't Properly Represented in Scientific Studies," *Slate*, July 28, 2010, www.slate.com/articles/health_and_science/medical_examiner/2010/07/drug_problem.single.html.

28 Elizabeth Claire, "How Is the RDA of Vitamin C Determined?" *Living Healthy 360*, January 22, 2009, www.livinghealthy360.com/index.php/how-is-rda-determined-26534.

29 Ibid.

30 Institute of Medicine, US Food and Nutrition Board, "What Are Dietary Reference Intakes?" in *Dietary Reference Intakes: A Risk Assessment Model for Establishing Upper Intake Levels for Nutrients* (Washington, DC: National Academies Press, 1998), www.ncbi.nlm.nih.gov/books/NBK45182.

31 Centers for Disease Control and Prevention, *Laboratory Medicine Best Practices*.

32 Ibid.

33 Shahram Shahangian and Susan R. Snyder, "Laboratory Medicine Quality Indicators: A Review of the Literature," *American Journal of Clinical Pathology* 131, no. 3 (March 2009): 418–31, http://ajcp.ascpjournals.org/content/131/3/418.full.

34 "How Reliable Is Laboratory Testing?"

35 Ibid.

CHAPTER 7

1 Rush University Medical Center, "New Criteria Proposed for Diagnosing Fibromyalgia," *Science Daily*, June 6, 2010, www.sciencedaily.com/releases/2010/05/100524143427.htm.

2 Ibid.

3 "Lyme Disease Data," CDC.

4 "Vector-Borne Disease Control," Virginia Department of Health Environmental Epidemiology, last updated June 5, 2013, www.vdh.virginia.gov/epidemiology/DEE/Vectorborne.

5 "Lyme Disease Data," Centers for Disease Control and Prevention, last updated September 16, 2013, www.cdc.gov/lyme/stats.

6 "Reported Cases of Lyme Disease by Year, United States, 1991–2004." DVBID: Disease Upward Climb, CDC LymeDisease. Oct. 24, 2005, http://www.cdc.gov/ncidod/dvbid/lyme/ldUpClimbLymeDis.htm.

7 "A History of Lyme Disease, Symptoms, Diagnosis, Treatment, and Prevention." National Institute of Allergy and Infectious Diseases, last updated October 9, 2012, www.niaid.nih.gov/topics/lymedisease/understanding/pages/intro.aspx.

8 "Ignorance of Tick-Borne Lyme Disease 'Costing Lives,'" BBC News, May 11, 2013, www.bbc.co.uk/news/health-22468181.

9 "Post-Treatment Lyme Disease Syndrome," Centers for Disease Control and Prevention, last updated February 7, 2013, www.cdc.gov/lyme/postLDS/index.html.

10 A. C. Steere, R. T. Schoen, and E. Taylor, "The Clinical Evolution of Lyme Arthritis," *Annals of Internal Medicine* 107, no. 5 (November 1987): 725–31, www.ncbi.nlm.nih.gov/pubmed/3662285.

11 J. J. Nocton et al., "Detection of Borrelia burgdorferi DNA by Polymerase Chain Reaction in Synovial Fluid from Patients with Lyme Arthritis," *New England Journal of Medicine* 330, no. 4 (January 27, 1994): 229–34, www.ncbi.nlm.nih.gov/pubmed/8272083.

12 ClinicalTrials.gov, US National Institutes of Health, accessed May 2013, http://clinicaltrials.gov/ct2/results?term=lyme.

13 A. M. Ercolini and S. D. Miller, "The Role of Infections in Autoimmune Disease," *Clinical & Experimental Immunology* 155, no. 1 (January 2009): 1–15, www.ncbi.nlm.nih.gov/pmc/articles/PMC2665673.

14 "Post-Treatment Lyme Disease Syndrome."

15 "Ignorance of Tick-Borne Lyme Disease 'Costing Lives,'" BBC.

16 Ibid.

17 Denise Mann, "Risk of Shingles Recurrence Is Low," WebMD, June 5, 2012, www.webmd.com/skin-problems-and-treatments/shingles/news/20120605/risk-shingles-recurrence-is-low.

18 S. Giovanoli et al., "Stress in Puberty Unmasks Latent Neuropathological Consequences of Prenatal Immune Activation in Mice," *Science* 339, no. 6123 (March 1, 2013): 1095–99, www.sciencemag.org/content/339/6123/1095.abstract?sid=a8d32de1-2adf-4052-89b8-2e1b6ce55fe0.

19 Emily Underwood, "One-Two Punch of Infection, Stress May Lead to Schizophrenia," *Science*NOW, February 28, 2013, http://news.sciencemag.org/sciencenow/2013/02/one-two-punch-of-infection-stress-may-lead-schizophrenia.

20 Ibid.

21 S. Campbell and G. MacQueen, "The Role of the Hippocampus in the Pathophysiology of Major Depression," *Journal of Psychiatry & Neuroscience* 29, no. 6 (November 2004): 417–26, www.ncbi.nlm.nih.gov/pmc/articles/PMC524959/#r28-2.

22 J. D. Bremner et al., "MRI-Based Measurement of Hippocampal Volume in Patients with Combat-Related Posttraumatic Stress Disorder," *American Journal of Psychiatry* 152, no. 7 (July 1995): 973–81, www.ncbi.nlm.nih.gov/pubmed/7793467.

23 A. J. McDermid, G. B. Rollman, and G. A. McCain, "Generalized Hypervigilance in Fibromyalgia: Evidence of Perceptual Amplification," *Pain* 66, nos. 2–3 (August 1996): 133–44, www.ncbi.nlm.nih.gov/pubmed/8880834.

24 Underwood, "One-Two Punch."

25 Kathleen A. Kendall-Tackett, "Physiological Correlates of Childhood Abuse: Chronic Hyperarousal in PTSD, Depression, and Irritable Bowel Syndrome," *Child Abuse & Neglect* 24, no. 6 (2000): 799–810, www.neurofeedbackclinic.ca/journals/ptsd/ptsd01.pdf.

26 N. J. Talley et al., "Gastrointestinal Tract Symptoms and Self-Reported Abuse: A Population-Based Study," *Gastroenterology* 107, no. 4 (October 1994): 1040–49, www.ncbi.nlm.nih.gov/pubmed/7926457.

27 Kendall-Tackett, "Physiological Correlates of Childhood Abuse."

28 Stephen Shuchter, Nancy Downs, and Sidney Zisook, *Biologically Informed Psychotherapy for Depression* (New York: Guilford Press, 1996); and R. M. Post, D. R. Rubinow, and J. C. Ballenger, "Conditioning and Sensitisation in the Longitudinal Course of Affective Illness," *British Journal of Psychiatry* 149 (August 1986): 191–201, www.ncbi.nlm.nih.gov/pubmed/3535979.

29 J. N. Briere and D. M. Elliot, "Immediate and Long-Term Impacts of Child Sexual Abuse," *Future of Children* 4 (Summer–Fall 1994): 54–69, http://futureofchildren.org/futureofchildren/publications/docs/04_02_02.pdf.

30 Judith Herman, *Trauma and Recovery* (New York: Basic Books, 1992), 96.

31 J. Leserman et al., "Sexual and Physical Abuse History in Gastroenterology Practice: How Types of Abuse Impact Health Status," *Psychosomatic Medicine* 58, no. 1 (January–February 1996): 4–15, www.ncbi.nlm.nih.gov/pubmed/8677288.

32 Ibid.

33 H. S. Resnick et al., "Effect of Previous Trauma on Acute Plasma Cortisol Level Following Rape," *American Journal of Psychiatry* 152, no. 11 (November 1995): 1675–77, www.ncbi.nlm.nih.gov/pubmed/7485635.

34 R. Yehuda, A. C. McFarlane, and A. Y. Shalev, "Predicting the Development of Posttraumatic Stress Disorder from the Acute Response to a Traumatic Event," *Biological Psychiatry* 44, no. 12 (December 15, 1998): 1305–13, www.ncbi.nlm.nih.gov/pubmed/9861473.

35 Thomas Insel, "Transforming Diagnosis," Director's Blog, National Institute of Mental Health, April 29, 2013, www.nimh.nih.gov/about/director/2013/transforming-diagnosis.shtml.

CHAPTER 8

1 R. C. Kessler, K. R. Merikangas, and P. S. Wang, "Prevalence, Comorbidity, and Service Utilization for Mood Disorders in the United States at the Beginning of the Twenty-First Century," *Annual Review of Clinical Psychology* 3 (2007): 137–58, www.ncbi.nlm.nih.gov/pubmed/17716051.

2 Institute of Medicine Report from the Committee on Advancing Pain Research, Care, and Education, *Relieving Pain in America: A Blueprint for Transforming Prevention, Care, Education, and Research* (Washington, DC: National Academies Press, 2011), http://books.nap.edu/openbook.php?record_id=13172&page=1.

3 World IBD Day 2011, accessed September 2013, http://worldibdday.com.

4 Mark Hyman, *The UltraMind Solution: Fix Your Broken Brain by Healing Your Body First* (New York: Scribner), Kindle edition, 172.

5 Annie Stuart, "Autoimmune Disease and RA," WebMD Rheumatoid Arthritis Health Center, last reviewed June 17, 2009, www.webmd.com/rheumatoid-arthritis/features/autoimmune-disease-and-ra.

6 "Sleeping Disorder Statistics," Statistic Brain, verified February 7, 2012, www.statisticbrain.com/sleeping-disorder-statistics.

7 "Greetings, Health Care Professional," American Sleep Apnea Association, accessed October 2013, www.sleepapnea.org/i-am-a-health-care-professional.html.

8 "65 Percent of American Adults Are Overweight and 31 Percent of Adults Are Obese and at Risk for Chronic Diseases," News-Medical.Net, June 11, 2004, www.news-medical.net/news/2004/06/11/2381.aspx.

9 S. M. Wilhelm, R. G. Rjater, and P. B. Kale-Pradhan, "Perils and Pitfalls of Long-Term Effects of Proton Pump Inhibitors," *Expert Review of Clinical Pharmacology* 6, no. 4 (July 2013): 443–51, www.medscape.com/viewarticle/809193.

10 J. Leuschen et al., "Association of Statin Use with Cataracts," *JAMA Ophthalmology*, September 19, 2013, www.ncbi.nlm.nih.gov/pubmed/24052188.

11 I. Mansi et al., "Statins and Musculoskeletal Conditions, Arthropathies, and Injuries," *JAMA Internal Medicine* 173, no. 14 (July 22, 2013): 1–10, www.ncbi.nlm.nih.gov/pubmed/23877079.

12 U. K. Sampson, M. F. Linton, and S. Fazio, "Are Statins Diabetogenic?" *Current Opinion in Cardiology* 26, no. 4 (July 2011): 342–47, www.ncbi.nlm.nih.gov/pmc/articles/PMC3341610.

13 Adebayao D. Djamason, "Is Non-Steroidal Anti-Inflammatory Drug (NSAID) Enteropathy Clinically More Important Than NSAID Gastropathy?" *Postgraduate Medical Journal* 82, no. 965 (March 2006): 186–91; I. Tacheci, P. Bradna, T. Douda, et al., "NSAID-Induced Enteropathy in Rheumatoid Arthritis Patients with Chronic Occult Gastrointestinal Bleeding," *Gastroenterology Research and Practice* 2013 (2013).

14 C. Brock, S. S. Olesen, A. E. Olesen, et al., "Opioid-Induced Bowel Dysfunction," *Drugs* 72, no. 14 (October 1, 2012): 1847–65; J. F. Scherrer, D. M. Svrakic, K. E. Freedland, et al., "Prescription Opioid Analgesics Increase the Risk of Depression," *Journal of General Internal Medicine* (October 29, 2013).

15 D. F. Kripke, R. D. Langer, L. E. Kline, "Hypnotics Associated with Mortality or Cancer: A Matched Cohort Study," *British Medical Journal* 2, no. 1 (February 27, 2012).

16 H. Pétursson, "The Benzodiazepine Withdrawal Syndrome," *Addiction* 89, no. 11 (November 1994): 1455–59, www.ncbi.nlm.nih.gov/pubmed/7841856.

17 R. H. Rahe and R. J. Arthur, "Life Change and Illness Studies: Past History and Future Directions," *Journal of Human Stress* 4, no. 1 (March 1978): 3–15, www.ncbi.nlm.nih.gov/pubmed/346993.

18 Hyman, *The UltraMind Solution.*

19 D. E. King et al., "Dietary Magnesium and C-Reactive Protein Levels," *Journal of the American College of Nutrition* 24, no. 3 (June 2005): 166–71, www.ncbi.nlm.nih.gov/pubmed/15930481.

20 "Dietary Supplement Fact Sheet: Magnesium," Office of Dietary Supplements, National Institutes of Health, last reviewed November 4, 2013, http://ods.od.nih.gov/factsheets/Magnesium-HealthProfessional.

21 M. F. Holick and T. C. Chen, "Vitamin D Deficiency: A Worldwide Problem with Health Consequences," *American Journal of Clinical Nutrition* 87, no. S4 (April 2008): S1080–S1086, http://ajcn.nutrition.org/content/87/4/1080S.full.

22 Barry Sears, *The Anti-Inflammation Zone* (New York: HarperCollins), Kindle edition, 1262–63.

23 Ibid.

24 Dani Cooper, "Motor Neurone Clue in Blue-Green Algae," ABC Science, September 26, 2013, www.abc.net.au/science/articles/2013/09/26/3856265.htm.

25 Barry Sears, *The Omega Rx Zone* (New York: HarperCollins, 2009), Kindle edition.

26 Sears, *The Anti-Inflammation Zone.*

27 Ibid.

28 Ibid.

29 Ibid.

30 Kathleen Doheny, "Choose Dark Chocolate for Health Benefits," WebMD, April 24, 2012, www.webmd.com/diet/news/20120424/pick-dark-chocolate-health-benefits.

31 K. J. Mukamal et al., "Tea Consumption and Mortality after Acute Myocardial Infarction," *Circulation* 105 (2002): 2476–81, http://circ.ahajournals.org/content/105/21/2476.full; and "Tea and Cardiovascular Health," Tea Guardian, accessed September 2013, http://teaguardian.com/tea-health/heart disease.html#.UknI0VOkeSo

32 S. Bhagwat, D. Haytowitz, and J. Holden, *USDA Database for the Flavonoid Content of Selected Foods: Release 3.1*, June 2013, www.ars.usda.gov/SP2UserFiles/Place/12354500/Data/Flav/Flav3-1.pdf.

33 H. A. Eyre, E. Papps, and B. T. Baune, "Treating Depression and Depression-like Behavior with Physical Activity: An Immune Perspective," *Front Psychiatry* 4, no. 3 (February 4, 2013): 3; R. A. Kohman et al., "Exercise Reduces Activation of Microglia Isolated from Hippocampus and Brain of Aged Mice," *Journal of Neuroinflammation* 10, no. 1 (September 18, 2013): 114; and K. M. Gerecke et al., "Exercise Protects

Against Chronic Restraint Stress-Induced Oxidative Stress in the Cortex and Hippocampus," *Brain Research* 1509 (May 6, 2013): 66–78.

34 Tom Venuto, *The Body Fat Solution* (New York: Penguin, 2009).

35 J. A. Astin et al., "Mind-Body Medicine: State of the Science, Implications for Practice," *Journal of the American Board of Family Medicine* 16, no. 2 (March 1, 2003): 131–47, www.jabfm.org/content/16/2/131.abstract?sid=346d3017-90b6-465b-8025-b0c4ae33b2ed.

36 M. A. Rosenkranz et al., "A Comparison of Mindfulness-Based Stress Reduction and an Active Control in Modulation of Neurogenic Inflammation," *Brain Behavior, and Immunity* 27, no. 1 (January 2013): 174–84, www.ncbi.nlm.nih.gov/pubmed/23092711.

37 D. A. Monti et al., "Changes in Cerebral Blood Flow and Anxiety Associated with an 8-Week Mindfulness Programme in Women with Breast Cancer," *Stress and Health* 28, no. 5 (December 2012): 397–407, www.ncbi.nlm.nih.gov/pubmed/23129559.

38 M. K. Leung et al., "Increased Gray Matter Volume in the Right Angular and Posterior Parahippocampal Gyri in Loving-Kindness Meditators, *Social Cognitive and Affective Neuroscience* 8, no. 1 (January 2013): 34–39, www.ncbi.nlm.nih.gov/pmc/articles/PMC3541494.

39 J. Younger et al., "Low-Dose Naltrexone for the Treatment of Fibromyalgia: Findings of a Small, Randomized, Double-Blind, Placebo-Controlled, Counterbalanced, Crossover Trial Assessing Daily Pain Levels," *Arthritis and Rheumatism* 65, no. 2 (February 2013): 529–38; P. Chopra and M. S. Cooper, "Treatment of Complex Regional Pain Syndrome (CRPS) Using Low Dose Naltrexone (LDN)," *Journal of Neuroimmune Pharmacology* 8, no. 3 (June 2013): 470–766; R. N. Donahue, P. J. McLaughlin, and I. S. Zagon, "Low-Dose Naltrexone Suppresses Ovarian Cancer and Exhibits Enhanced Inhibition in Combination with Cisplatin," *Experimental Biology and Medicine (Maywood)* 236, no. 7 (July 2011): 883–95; and N. Brown and J. Panksepp, "Low-Dose Naltrexone for Disease Prevention and Quality of Life," *Medical Hypotheses* 72, no. 3 (March 2009): 333–37.

40 C. Sun et al., "Neuroprotective Effect of Minocycline in a Rat Model of Branch Retinal Vein Occlusion," *Experimental Eye Research* 113 (August 2013): 105–16; R. A. Kohman et al., "Effects of Minocycline on Spatial Learning, Hippocampal Neurogenesis and Microglia in Aged and Adult Mice," *Behavioural Brain Research* 242 (April 2013): 17–24; and M. Watabe et al., "Minocycline, a Microglial Inhibitor, Reduces 'Honey Trap' Risk in Human Economic Exchange," *Scientific Reports* 3 (2013): 1685.

41 J. M. Saavedra, "Angiotensin II AT(1) Receptor Blockers as Treatments for Inflammatory Brain Disorders," *Clinical Science (London)* 123, no. 10 (November 2012): 567–90; R. Timaru-Kast et al., "Delayed Inhibition of Angiotensin II Receptor Type 1 Reduces Secondary Brain Damage and Improves Functional Recovery after Experimental Brain Trauma," *Critical Care Medicine* 40, no. 3 (March 2012): 935–44; and J. Benicky et al., "Angiotensin II AT1 Receptor Blockade Ameliorates Brain Inflammation," *Neuropsychopharmacology* 36, no. 4 (March 2011): 857–70.

RESOURCES

1 Mark Hyman, UltraMetabolism: The Simple Plan for Automatic Weight Loss (New York: Atria Books), 143.

2 J. G. Montoya et al., "Randomized Clinical Trial to Evaluate the Efficacy and Safety of Valganciclovir in a Subset of Patients with Chronic Fatigue Syndrome," Journal of Medical Virology 85, no. 12 (December 2013): 2101–09, www.ncbi.nlm.nih.gov/pubmed/23959519.

Acknowledgments

Like many projects in life, writing a book, especially a book on medical issues, requires a team effort. I am a clinician and a teacher, and Donna Beech is a gifted writer. This book has been a true collaboration between us, and I am grateful for her talent and contributions in bringing this project to completion. Thank you, Donna, for "getting it" and for being patient while I fretted over numerous rewrites, making sure that we got the medicine and the science right.

For their insights and support, I also want to thank my colleagues and friends José Apud, MD; Bernardo Hirschman, MD; Michael Diamond, MD; Michael Lumpkin, PhD; John Reed, MD; Lisa Lillienfield, MD; Jodi Brayton, LCSW, MSW; Nan Kinder, RN; and Robin Harris, RN. Your contributions to our study group were the seeds from which this book took root.

I am also grateful to my colleagues who reviewed this book's factual and technical content: Jay Shah, MD; John Reed, MD; Joseph Helms, MD; Brian Berman, MD; Adi Harimati, PhD; José Apud, MD; Emily Ratner, MD; and Rudy Bauer, PhD. I asked a lot of these very busy people, whose comments and recommendations significantly improved the book.

I also am indebted to Linda Pierce, whose skills as a librarian brought order to the chaos of well over 1,000 research publications that needed to be referenced and cataloged.

I also want to thank my friends Richard Rossi; John Reed, MD; and Alan Cheuse. Richard not only encouraged me to take on this project, but he and his wife, Lisa, also provided the refuge of their home on Block Island for research and writing. My dear friend and colleague John Reed and I spent many years working together, finding better ways to help our patients. Alan Cheuse, a gifted writer and teacher, read the early chapters of the book and gave me the great gift of introducing me to his agent, Michael V. Carlisle. Thank you, Alan.

Michael V. Carlisle and his Inkwell Management colleagues guided this book throughout the publication process and provided invaluable support along the way. I am also indebted to Rodale and publisher Mary Ann Naples for believing in the value of this book—and to Alex Postman, an outstanding editor. Alex recognized we were shy a critical chapter, and the book is much better because of her.

Some of my greatest teachers have been my patients—several of whom agreed to be interviewed for this book and allowed their stories to be told in the hopes that others might benefit. I am deeply grateful for the trust that all of my patients have placed in me in allowing me to care for them and for all that they have taught me about health and healing. Thank you.

No project can be created without a solid foundation. In my life, my wife, Fran, is that foundation. She is wise, intelligent, insightful, and a source of inspiration, love, and support in my life. Thank you, Fran.

Index

C

D

E

F

G

H

I

J

K

L

M

N

O

P

R

S

T

V

W

X

Z